NEW DEVELOPMENTS IN MEDICAL RESEARCH

AN ESSENTIAL GUIDE TO ASTAXANTHIN

DIETARY SOURCES, PROPERTIES AND HEALTH BENEFITS

NEW DEVELOPMENTS IN MEDICAL RESEARCH

Additional books and e-books in this series can be found on Nova's website under the Series tab.

BIOCHEMISTRY RESEARCH TRENDS

Additional books and e-books in this series can be found on Nova's website under the Series tab.

NEW DEVELOPMENTS IN MEDICAL RESEARCH

AN ESSENTIAL GUIDE TO ASTAXANTHIN

DIETARY SOURCES, PROPERTIES AND HEALTH BENEFITS

PAUL A. MELBORNE
EDITOR

nova
science publishers
New York

Library of Congress Cataloging-in-Publication Data

ISBN: 978-1-53615-571-6

Published by Nova Science Publishers, Inc. † New York

CONTENTS

PREFACE

An Essential Guide to Astaxanthin: Dietary Sources, Properties and Health Benefits begins with a review of published studies regarding the efficacy and application of natural astaxanthin in aquaculture and human health, respectively.

Next, to help in optimizing astaxanthin production, the changes of pigments (including chlorophyll and carotenoids) and astaxanthin geometrical isomers were elucidated during the incubation in H. pluvialis under environmental stresses. Changes in photosynthetic behaviors and photoprotective mechanisms during astaxanthin accumulation were clarified.

In the closing chapter, the authors review methods for Z-isomerization of astaxanthin and subsequent changes in the physicochemical properties and functionalities.

Chapter 1 - An Essential Guide to Astaxanthin: Dietary Sources, Properties and Health Benefits begins with a review of published studies regarding the efficacy and application of natural astaxanthin in aquaculture and human health, respectively. Next, to help in optimizing astaxanthin production, the changes of pigments (including chlorophyll and carotenoids) and astaxanthin geometrical isomers were elucidated during the incubation in H. pluvialis under environmental stresses. Changes in photosynthetic behaviors and photoprotective mechanisms during astaxanthin accumulation were clarified. In the closing chapter, the authors review methods for Z-isomerization of astaxanthin and subsequent changes in the physicochemical properties and functionalities.

Chapter 2 - Astaxanthin has important applications in the nutraceutical, cosmetic, food and feed industries due to its extraordinary antioxidant capability. Unicellular green alga *Haematococcus pluvialis* is recognized as one of the most promising producer of astaxanthin in nature due to its exceptional ability to accumulate large amounts of astaxanthin under environmental stresses. In this review, the terms and concepts of the cell forms of *H. pluvialis* at various cell cycles stages are re-defined in an effort to avoid confusion and awkward phrasing. The changes of pigments (including chlorophyll and carotenoids) and astaxanthin geometrical isomers are elucidated during the incubation in *H. pluvialis* under environmental stresses. Changes in photosynthetic behaviors and photoprotective mechanisms during astaxanthin accumulation are clarified. The astaxanthin metabolic process and regulation are elucidated through analyzing the relationship between astaxanthin biosynthesis and chlororespiration, photorespiration, fatty acid biosynthesis. Meanwhile, an unknown bioactive substance by *H. pluvialis*, which can feed back influence cell growth and transformation from motile cells into non-motile cells, has been revealed. Cultivation of *H. pluvialis* for astaxanthin production in phototrophic, heterotrophic, mixotrophic and heterotrophic-phototrophic culture modes are presented. The biological contamination control during cultivation of *H. pluvialis* is analyzed. In the near future, the genome sequencing and genetic toolbox development will affect significantly future advancement in *H. pluvialis* and astaxanthin biosynthesis research. Mass cultivation of *H. pluvialis* is already physically and economically feasible and profitable, and this industry is bound to expand.

Chapter 3 - Astaxanthin, a pigment that belongs to the family of xanthophylls, has a large number of geometric isomers due to the presence of numerous conjugated double bonds in the molecule. A number of studies have addressed that *Z*-isomers of astaxanthin would have a higher bioavailability and show a higher antioxidant capacity than the all-*E*-

isomer. Hence, it is important to understand efficient *Z*-isomerization method for (all-*E*)-astaxanthin. Furthermore, very recently, several experiments have shown that the *Z*-isomerization of carotenoids including astaxanthin induced the changes in the physicochemical properties such as solubility and crystallinity. It is considered that the changes in physicochemical properties of carotenoids by the *Z*-isomerization would be closely involved in the changes of the functionalities, and an accurate understanding of the relationship could contribute to fully exerting the health benefits of astaxanthin. The objective of this contribution is to review methods for *Z*-isomerization of astaxanthin and subsequent changes in the physicochemical properties and functionalities.

In: An Essential Guide to Astaxanthin ISBN: 978-1-53615-571-6
Editor: Paul A. Melborne

Chapter 1

EFFICACY AND APPLICATION OF THE NATURAL ASTAXANTHIN

Hu Li[1,2], Jianguo Liu[1,2,3,*] and Ling Li[1,2]
[1]CAS Key Laboratory of Experimental Marine Biology,
Center for Ocean Mega-Science, Institute of Oceanology,
Chinese Academy of Sciences, Qingdao, China
[2]Laboratory for Marine Biology and Biotechnology,
Qingdao National Laboratory for Marine Science and Technology,
Aoshanwei Town, Jimo, Qingdao, China
[3]National-Local Joint Engineering Research Center for
Haematococcus pluvialis and Astaxanthin Products,
Yunnan Alphy Biotech Co., Ltd., Chuxiong, China

ABSTRACT

To date, a number of articles have been published on the efficacy and application of the natural astaxanthin. In aquaculture, the shrimp postlarvae fed with natural astaxanthin diets showed significantly higher

* Corresponding Author's E-mail: jgliu@qdio.ac.cn.

growth performance and astaxanthin content. The supplement of *H. pluvialis* natural astaxanthin had significant dose-depended effects on the accumulation of carotenoid in ovary, hepatopancreas, carapace and epidermis of crabs. Similarly, feeding trials in rotifers with the defatted *H. pluvialis* meal (DHPM) showed that DHPM addition is beneficial for rotifer growth, and enhance the nutritional quality of the rotifers. Meanwhile, supplement of the natural astaxanthin in rainbow trout cultivation also showed a similar improvement of the meat color and quality. In the field of human health, the high anti-oxidant capacity and polar features of astaxanthin make it an amazing nutraceutical for favorable applications. The natural astaxanthin can improve the memory of middle-aged BALB/c mice. Our feeding trial in APP/PS1 mice (the Alzheimer's Disease-AD model mice) suggested that natural astaxanthin has some beneficial effects on the pathology of AD mice. Besides, an obviously preventive effect of astaxanthin on AKI in the tested Wistar rats was also observed. This chapter reviews the published studies about the efficacy and application of the natural astaxanthin in aquaculture and human health, respectively.

APPLICATION IN AQUACULTURE

Aquaculture animals lack the ability to synthesize carotenoids, the pigments must be included in their feeds. Astaxanthin, a carotenoid naturally synthesized in some plants, algae, and bacteria, is amassed by many fishes, crustaceans, and birds through food chains in nature. Recently astaxanthin are used gainfully in aquaculture as feed additive and dietary supplement. As a dietary supplement, astaxanthin not only is a source of pigment in the feed of aquaculture animals (salmon, trout and shrimp, etc.), but also has been reported as having anti-aging, anti-inflammatory, and sun proofing properties, positively influence growth, reproductive performance, and boost immune system in aquaculture animals. There are many reports about the beneficial dietary supplement of natural astaxanthin from *Haematococcus pluvialis* for live feed organisms, shrimps, crabs and fishes in aquaculture.

Live Feed Organisms

The rotifer and cladoceran are useful live feed organisms for the rearing of fish, shrimp and shellfish larvae in aquaculture. Our feeding trials in live feed organism rotifers (*Brachionus plicatilis*) with the defatted *H. pluvialis* meal (DHPM, containing 0.5% residual astaxanthin) showed that the addition of DHPM is beneficial for their growth (Figure 1) and enhanced the nutritional quality of them as first feed for aquaculture (Li et al., 2019). It was found that the DHPM was accumulated in the rotifer gut after rotifers were fed with DHPM (Figure 2A). The total carotenoid and astaxanthin concentrations of live feed organisms after feeding on DHPM increased. The same result was observed in another live feed organism *Moina macrocopa* (the *Moina macrocopa* gut turned red and their nutritional quality were enhanced after fed with DHPM) (Figure 2C).

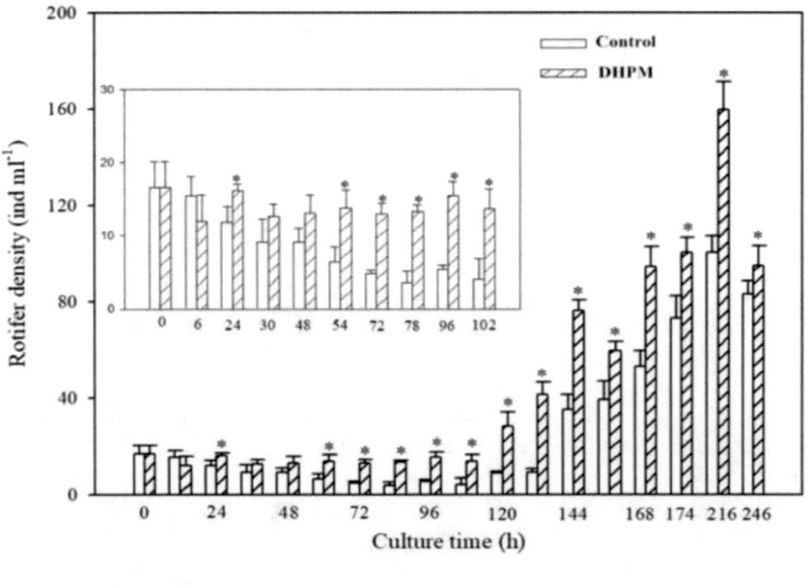

Figure 1. Changes of rotifer (*Brachionus plicatilis*) density (the number of rotifers per ml) during culturing for 246 h in the control (0 mg l^{-1} DHPM) and treatment (125 mg l^{-1} DHPM) groups (Inset shows growth from 0 to 102 h). Means ± SD of four replicates are presented (n = 4). (*$P < 0.05$, compared to the respective control).

Furthermore, a recent study (Johnston et al., 2018) also suggested that after supplemented with astaxanthin oleoresin extracted from *H. pluvialis*, *Brachionus manjavacas* rotifer cultures reached significantly higher population densities and maintained them for longer. After fed with astaxanthin, rotifers enhanced their resistance to oxidative stress. They concluded that natural astaxanthin can be used to improve the productivity and stability of rotifer mass cultures by increasing oxidative stress resistance and enhance the nutritional content of rotifers for larval fish.

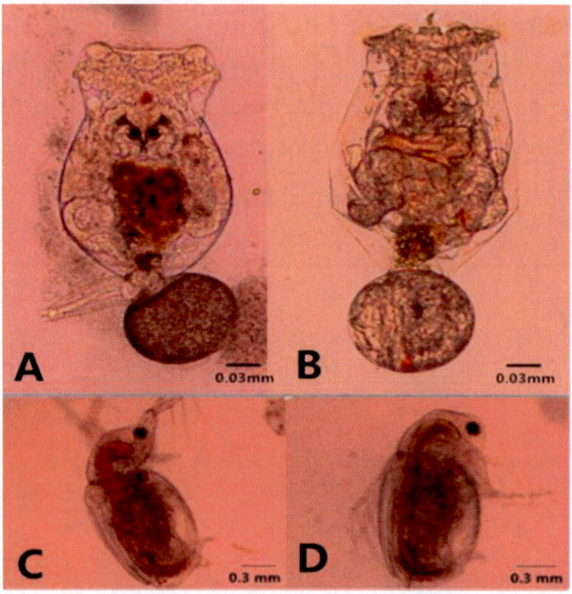

Figure 2. A comparison of the rotifer (*B. plicatilis*) (A, B) and *M. macrocopa* (C, D) fed with DHPM (A, C) and without DHPM (B, D). DHPM were accumulated in the rotifer (A) and *M. macrocopa* (C) gut, respectively.

Shrimps

Astaxanthin is a beneficial dietary supplement in shrimp farming. Synthetic astaxanthin (S-Ast) is significantly inferior to algal-based astaxanthin as an antioxidant and may not be suitable as a human or animal nutraceutical supplement (Capelli et al., 2013). However, the different effects of synthetic astaxanthin (S-Ast) and natural astaxanthin (N-Ast) on the postlarvae is unclear. Chien et al., (2005) found that the both N-Ast-fed and S-Ast-fed prawns (*Marsupenaeus japonicus)* had significantly higher survival rates than the no-Ast prawns. When subjected to low dissolved oxygen stress, no-Ast prawns had higher oxygen consumption rate (OCR) and shorter survival time (ST) than the prawns fed the astaxanthin diets (N-Ast and S-Ast). Recently, our results indicated that postlarvae given N-Ast had significantly higher growth performance (Figure 3) and astaxanthin content (Figure 4) (Liu et al., 2018). Although there were different ratios of astaxanthin optical isomers in the diets, there was a similar optical isomer content in juvenile shrimp (Figure 4D). The cis/trans astaxanthin ratio in N-Ast90 were the highest among all groups (Figure 4B). These results suggested that an epimerase may exist *in vivo* and that an appropriate level of botanical astaxanthin in diets was approximately 90 ppm for *L. vannamei* postlarvae (Liu et al., 2018).

Besides, Niu et al., (2012) compared the effects of astaxanthin, canthaxanthin and cholesterol on *Penaeus monodon* growth performance and antioxidant capacity. They concluded that astaxanthin was better than canthaxanthin as the dietary carotenoid source in the commercial diet of *P. monodon*, and the supplement of cholesterol could positively enhance the efficiency of astaxanthin and canthaxanthin.

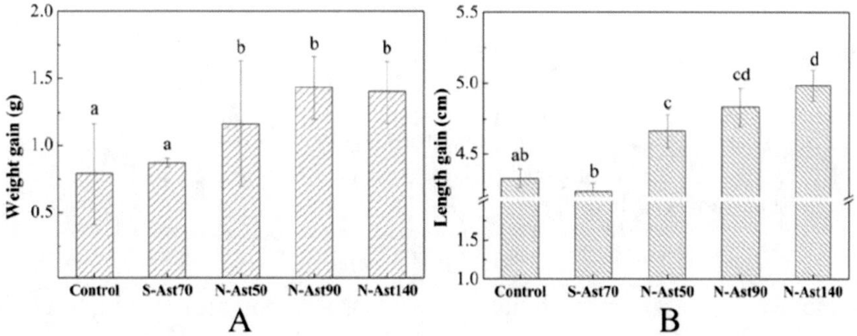

Source: Liu et al., 2018.

Figure 3. The weight and length gains of *L. vannamei* postlarvae after a 35-day feeding trial. Data with different letters (a, b, c, and d) are significantly different ($P < 0.05$, n = 30).

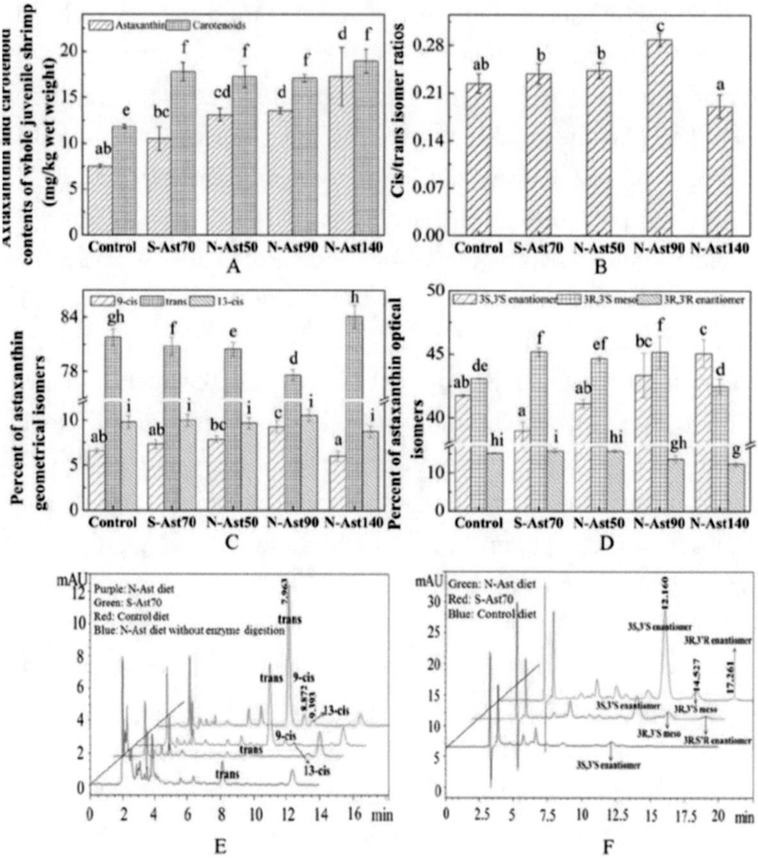

Source: Liu et al., 2018.

Figure 4. The carotenoid and astaxanthin contents (A), cis/trans isomer ratios (B), astaxanthin geometrical isomer percentages (C), astaxanthin optical isomer percentages (D), HPLC chromatograms of three diets using a silica column (E) and HPLC chromatograms of diets using a chiral column (F), in *Litopenaeus vannamei* postlarvae after a 35-day feeding trial. The significant differences are indicated by different superscripts (a, b, c, d, e and f) ($P < 0.05$, n = 3).

In the study of Ju et al., (2012), the effects of partial replacement of fishmeal by a defatted microalgae meal (DMM, containing 40.3% crude protein, 0.9% crude lipid and 0.05% astaxanthin) in a shrimp diet. After an 8-week feeding trial, shrimp fed DMM showed a significantly higher growth rate than the shrimp fed the control diet ($P < 0.05$). Besides, shrimp fed DMM-added diets appeared redder and contained higher free and esterified astaxanthins than shrimp fed the control diet.

Their results indicated that DMM could be a valuable alternative protein and pigmentation ingredient in shrimp feed. Astaxanthin-fed shrimps not only increased their survival rate, but also their resistance to *Vibrio parahaemolyticus*. Chuchird et al., (2015) found that the immune parameters, total hemocyte count (THC), phagocytosis activity, phenoloxidase (PO) activity, and superoxide dismutase (SOD) activity of astaxanthin-fed shrimps were significantly improved compared with the control shrimps (no astaxanthin).

Another 25-days experiment was conducted to evaluate the effects of dietary *H. pluvialis* on growth, survival, immune response and stress tolerance ability of post-larval *L. vannamei* (Xie et al., 2018). Post-larval white shrimp were fed five isoenergic and isonitrogenous diets containing grade levels of *H. pluvialis* (0, 1.7, 3.3, 6.7 and 13.3 g kg^{-1} diet, respectively). Their results indicated that 3.3 g *H. pluvialis* kg^{-1} diet increased the survival rate of post-larval white shrimp. After the acute salinity stress, survival of shrimp fed 6.7 g *H. pluvialis* kg^{-1} diet was significant higher than the control ($P < 0.05$), and the total antioxidant capacity was increased with the increasing dietary *H. pluvialis* levels. The malonaldehyde (MDA) contents in whole body decreased with the increasing dietary *H. pluvialis* levels before and after the salinity stress. After the salinity stress, relative mRNA levels of anti-oxidative related genes and immune related genes decreased with the dietary *H. pluvialis* level increased to 3.3 g kg^{-1}. Based on above results, they concluded that the optimal level of *H. pluvialis* was 3.3-6.7 g kg^{-1} diet (100-200 mg astaxanthin kg^{-1} diet) for *L. vannamei*.

Astaxanthin can block the bioaccumulation of toxin in crayfish. The crayfish, *Procambarus clarkia* (Girard, 1852), were cultured under microcystin-LR stress (0.025 mg l^{-1}) and were fed with fodders containing astaxanthin (0, 3, 6, 9, and 12 mg g^{-1}) for 8 weeks in glass tanks. Accumulations of microcystin-LR were measured in different organs of *P. clarkii*. The results suggested that astaxanthin could significantly improve the survival rate and specific growth rate of *P. clarkii* ($P < 0.05$).

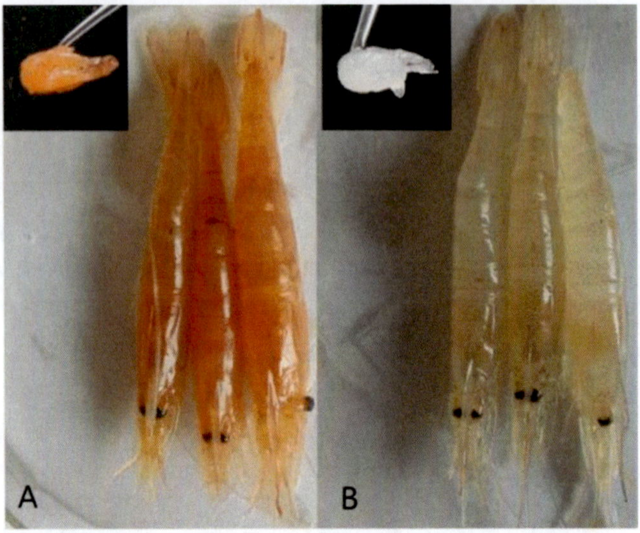

Source: Su F., 2018.

Figure 5. Representatives of the variety (A) and the conventional (B) *E. carinicauda*. They showed a distinct color difference in external characteristic and the inset was a cross-section view from the abdominal muscle from each shrimp.

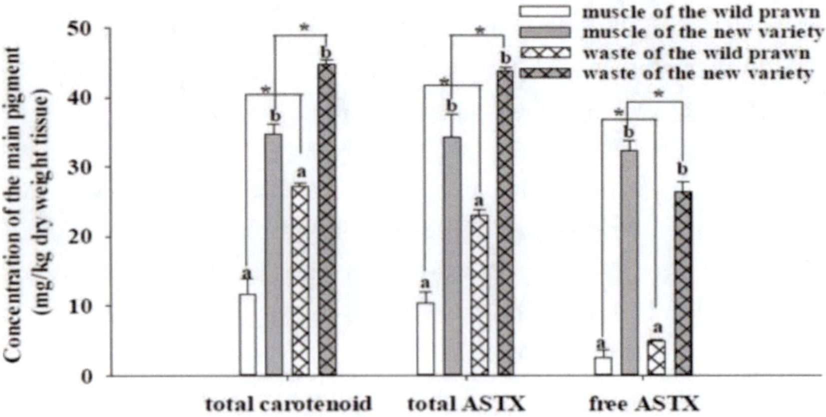

Source: Zhang et al., 2018.

Figure 6. The concentration (mean ± SD, n = 3) of total carotenoid, total astaxanthin (ASTX) and free ASTX in different tissues in the wild and the new variety of *E. carinicauda*. Different letters above the bars indicate significant differences between the wild and the new variety in the same tissue type and asterisk indicate significant differences between the muscle and the waste in the same prawn type ($P < 0.05$).

Table 1. Effects of dietary *H. pluvialis* powder on color values of ovaries, hepatopancreas and carapace of adult female *E. sinensis* (Data are presented as mean ± SE. Values within the same row with different letters mean significant difference ($P < 0.05$))

Items	Diet 1	Diet 2	Diet 3	Diet 4
Ovaries				
L^*	73.79 ± 0.63^a	67.19 ± 0.57^b	61.90 ± 0.43^c	61.17 ± 1.00^c
a^*	17.66 ± 0.92^b	23.61 ± 0.39^a	23.31 ± 0.69^a	24.20 ± 0.64^a
b^*	47.99 ± 1.00^a	40.45 ± 0.56^b	34.06 ± 0.94^c	32.60 ± 1.17^c
Hepatopancreas				
L^*	37.03 ± 1.82	37.90 ± 5.47	36.45 ± 4.86	32.92 ± 2.48
a^*	4.47 ± 0.67^b	5.17 ± 0.78^b	8.61 ± 0.48^a	6.24 ± 0.47^b
b^*	9.83 ± 0.94^b	11.14 ± 1.87^b	17.05 ± 2.06^a	12.70 ± 0.85^{ab}
Carapace				
L^*	68.38 ± 0.49^a	66.43 ± 0.50^{ab}	62.07 ± 0.62^c	65.70 ± 1.1^b
a^*	14.12 ± 0.46^c	15.85 ± 0.45^{bc}	18.68 ± 0.53^a	17.29 ± 1.12^{ab}
b^*	38.21 ± 1.25	37.14 ± 0.53	37.12 ± 0.92	37.22 ± 0.69

Source: Long et al., 2017.

Table 2. Effects of dietary H. pluvialis powder levels on serum antioxidant indices of adult female *E. sinensis* (Data are presented as mean ± SE. Values within the same row with different letters mean significant difference ($P < 0.05$))

Items	Diet 1	Diet 2	Diet 3	Diet 4
TAC (U ml^{-1})	8.05 ± 0.37	7.05 ± 0.30	8.00 ± 0.30	7.36 ± 0.47
SOD (U l^{-1})	39.40 ± 1.00	38.44 ± 0.75	41.06 ± 1.16	38.91 ± 0.78
CAT (U ml^{-1})	1.17 ± 0.04^{c}	1.82 ± 0.08^{b}	2.36 ± 0.24^{a}	1.93 ± 0.05^{b}
GPX (100 U ml^{-1})	23.03 ± 0.69^{b}	25.83 ± 0.84^{a}	26.29 ± 1.00^{a}	25.83 ± 0.48^{a}
GR (U l^{-1})	59.16 ± 3.15	59.49 ± 2.02	53.05 ± 4.82	52.52 ± 3.07
NO (µmol l^{-1})	10.83 ± 0.46^{c}	20.95 ± 1.99^{b}	23.96 ± 1.78^{ab}	28.15 ± 2.46^{a}
MDA (nmol ml^{-1})	6.18 ± 0.15^{a}	5.00 ± 0.14^{b}	4.24 ± 0.15^{c}	4.26 ± 0.08^{c}

Source: Long et al., 2017.

Table 3. Effects of dietary *H. pluvialis* powder levels on antioxidant indices in hepatopancreas of adult female *E. sinensis* (Data are presented as mean ± SE. Values within the same row with different letters mean significant difference ($P < 0.05$))

Items	Diet 1	Diet 2	Diet 3	Diet 4
TAC (U mg^{-1} protein)	2.44 ± 0.12	2.50 ± 0.15	2.30 ± 0.15	2.07 ± 0.12
SOD (U mg^{-1} protein)	6.04 ± 0.27	5.48 ± 0.31	6.12 ± 0.55	5.12 ± 0.38
GPX (U g^{-1} protein)	50.88 ± 2.58^{b}	67.63 ± 2.77^{a}	68.04 ± 2.60^{a}	55.08 ± 4.01^{b}
GR (U g^{-1} protein)	7.74 ± 0.45^{a}	5.23 ± 0.75^{c}	7.05 ± 0.58^{ab}	5.75 ± 0.55^{bc}
NO (µmol g^{-1} protein)	1.98 ± 0.07^{a}	1.65 ± 0.07^{b}	1.63 ± 0.05^{b}	1.47 ± 0.07^{b}
MDA (nmol mg^{-1} protein)	2.00 ± 0.11^{a}	2.17 ± 0.10^{a}	1.66 ± 0.10^{b}	1.43 ± 0.13^{b}

Source: Long et al., 2017.

Table 4. Effects of dietary *H. pluvialis* powder on proximate composition (% wet weight) in ovaries, hepatopancreas and muscle of adult female *E. sinensis* (Data are presented as mean ± SE. Values within the same row with different letters mean significant difference (P < 0.05))

Items	Diet 1	Diet 2	Diet 3	Diet 4
Ovaries				
Moisture	50.75 ± 0.72^{ab}	51.69 ± 0.55^{a}	50.28 ± 0.18^{ab}	49.69 ± 0.59^{b}
Crude protein	28.58 ± 0.07^{b}	28.18 ± 0.29^{b}	27.81 ± 0.56^{b}	29.79 ± 0.26^{a}
Crude lipid	14.73 ± 0.68	13.81 ± 0.66	14.40 ± 0.26	14.83 ± 0.33
Ash	1.82 ± 0.02	1.88 ± 0.10	1.78 ± 0.06	1.89 ± 0.19
Hepatopancreas				
Moisture	53.25 ± 0.44	52.87 ± 1.15	52.70 ± 0.89	52.45 ± 0.57
Crude protein	10.45 ± 0.67	10.93 ± 0.86	10.63 ± 0.98	9.88 ± 0.43
Crude lipid	31.71 ± 0.80	31.64 ± 0.89	30.65 ± 0.79	31.45 ± 0.92
Ash	1.40 ± 0.10^{ab}	1.21 ± 0.18^{b}	1.13 ± 0.13^{b}	1.71 ± 0.01^{a}
Muscle				
Moisture	78.42 ± 0.24^{ab}	79.49 ± 0.50^{a}	77.59 ± 0.41^{bc}	77.04 ± 0.50^{c}
Crude protein	17.65 ± 0.19^{b}	16.44 ± 0.13^{c}	17.94 ± 0.27^{ab}	18.50 ± 0.15^{a}
Crude lipid	1.06 ± 0.01^{a}	1.00 ± 0.02^{b}	1.08 ± 0.02^{a}	0.93 ± 0.02^{c}
Ash	1.87 ± 0.04	1.80 ± 0.04	1.72 ± 0.03	1.86 ± 0.07

Source: Long et al., 2017.

The dietary astaxanthin supplement seemed to block the bioaccumulation of microcystin-LR in the hepatopancreas and ovaries of *P. clarkii* to some extent ($P < 0.05$). Astaxanthin content of 9-12 mg g^{-1} in fodder can be a practical and economic choice (An et al., 2018). Astaxanthin was a protector of nitrite stress in shrimps. Díaz et al., (2014) investigated the effects of astaxanthin feed supplementation and environmental nitrite stress on postlarvae of *Pleoticus muelleri* under culture conditions. For all astaxanthin feed treatments, shrimps exhibited strong 1,1-diphenyl-2-picrylhydrazyl (DPPH) scavenging activity; however, shrimp fed with 100 mg kg^{-1} of diet and 300 mg kg^{-1} of diet showed the greatest activity to quench DPPH (62 and 59%, respectively) with respect to 0 mg kg^{-1} of diet (43%). They concluded that astaxanthin acts as a protector of nitrite stress in *P. muelleri*.

The ridgetail white prawn (*Exopalaemon carinicauda*) is an important economic species in China. Recently, a new variety with orangered color was found (Figure 5) (Su F., 2018; Zhang et al., 2018). In order to know the molecular basis and evaluate the potential nutrition value of the variety of this species, some studies were carried out by Zhang et al. (2018). They found that the higher concentration of free astaxanthin existed in the new variety which might cause the color variation. The concentration of total astaxanthin in muscle and waste of the new variety was 3.3 and 1.9 fold higher than that in natural prawn under the same culture condition (Figure 6). The predominant geometric and optical isomers of astaxanthin in muscle of the new variety were identified as all-trans and 3S, 3'S astaxanthin. This is the first report of astaxanthin-enriched *E. carinicauda*, which also provides an alternative source of natural astaxanthin and the possibility for improving the nutrition value in this species.

Crabs

The green algae *H. pluvialis* is an important natural astaxanthin producer, and natural astaxanthin is stable, mostly esterified, generally in the "all-trans" form and can be well-utilized by crabs.

Our team investigated the effects of dietary supplementation of *H. pluvialis* (rich in natural astaxanthin) powder on coloration, ovarian development and antioxidation capacity of adult female Chinese mitten crab, *Eriocheir sinensis* (Long et al., 2017). And four experimental diets were formulated to contain 0, 0.2%, 0.4% and 0.6% of *H. pluvialis* powder (defined as D1-D4, short for Diet 1~Diet 4). The results showed that dietary *H. pluvialis* powder had no significant effects on survival, gonadosomatic index (GSI) and hepatosomatic index (HSI) ($P > 0.05$). The redness (a*) of ovaries and carapace (Figure 7) as well as the contents of total carotenoid and astaxanthin in ovaries, hepatopancreas and carapace increased significantly with increasing dietary *H. pluvialis* powder, while a decreasing trend was found for the lightness (L*) and yellowness (b*) of ovaries; the highest and the lowest a* and b* of hepatopancreas were found for D3 and D1, respectively (Table 1). For antioxidant and immune parameters, crabs fed diets containing 0.4% of *H. pluvialis* cell powder had the highest levels of catalase (CAT), glutathione peroxidase (GPX), peroxidase (POD), hemocyanin (Hc) and γ-glutamyl transpeptidase (γ-GT) in the serum, while there was a significant decrease for the content of malondialdehyde (MDA) in serum (Table 2), as well as in the levels of nitric oxide (NO), MDA and acid phosphatase (ACP) in hepatopancreas (Table 3).

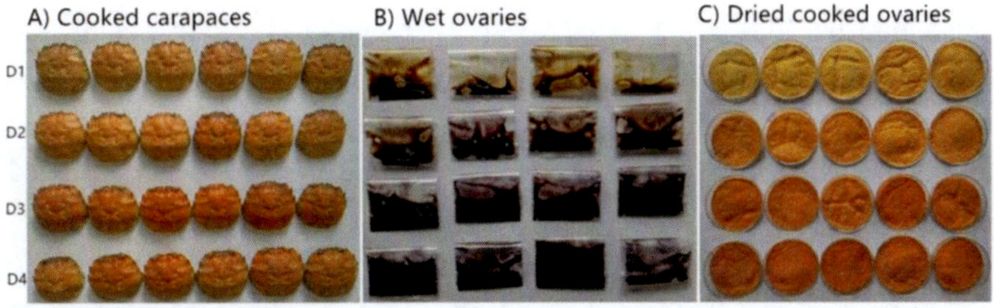

Source: Long et al., 2017.

Figure 7. Color of cooked carapaces (A), wet ovaries (B) and dried cooked ovaries (C) of adult female *E. sinensis* fed experimental diets for 60 days.

Dietary *H. pluvialis* powder had significant effects on the contents of moisture and crude protein in ovaries and muscle as well as hepatopancreatic ash level (Table 4). In conclusion, dietary *H. pluvialis* powder had no significant effect on ovarian development, but enhanced coloration, antioxidation capacity and improved protein content in ovaries and muscle of female *E. sinensis*. Wu et al., (2017) also studied the effects of dietary supplementation of *H. pluvialis* powder on gonadal development, coloration and antioxidant capacity of adult male Chinese mitten crab (*E. sinensis*). Their results suggested that the optimal dietary natural astaxanthin level was around 40 mg kg^{-1} diets.

Fishes

A high intake of astaxanthin through some fishes, is considered beneficial for human health because of their antioxidant activity. Sea animal that has the highest concentration of this astaxanthin is salmon. There were many researches about pigmentation, uptake and deposition of the natural astaxanthin in salmons.

Arai et al., (1987) had studied the pigmentation of juvenile coho salmon (*Oncorhynchus kisutch*) with carotenoid ((3R,3′ R)-astaxanthin diester as a main carotenoid) oil extracted from Antarctic krill (*Euphausia superba*). Their results suggested that the marked pigmentation was observed in fish flesh after fishes were reared on diets containing 7.2 mg astaxanthin per 100 g diet for 4 weeks. Bjerkeng et al., (2000) compared the apparent astaxanthin digestibility coefficients (ADC) and carotenoid compositions of the muscle, liver, whole kidney and plasma in Atlantic salmon (*Salmo salar*) and Atlantic halibut (*Hippoglossus hippoglossus*) fed a *diet* supplemented with 66 mg astaxanthin kg^{-1} dry matter for 112 days. They concluded that the higher ADC of astaxanthin in halibut than Atlantic salmon may be explained by *lower feed intake* in halibut, and the lower retention of astaxanthin by a higher capacity to transform astaxanthin metabolically.

Above feeding trials in Chinese mitten crabs showed that the dietary supplement of the *H. pluvialis* astaxanthin had significant effects on the accumulation of carotenoid in ovary, hepatopancreas, carapace and epidermis of Chinese mitten crabs. There was a clear dose-effect relationship between the carotenoid content deposited in tissues and the addition amount of *H. pluvialis* astaxanthin in feed.

In addition, there are many studies on the uptake and deposition of astaxanthin in rainbow trout. For example, Ytres tøyl et al., (2007) compared the effects of intraperitoneal (IP) injection astaxanthin and feeding astaxanthin diets on uptake of astaxanthin in plasma, muscle, kidney and liver of rainbow trout. They concluded that a more rapid and higher uptake of astaxanthin in plasma, muscle, kidney and liver of rainbow trout took place after IP compared to when astaxanthin was fed via the diet. Bowen et al., (2002) studied the deposition of natural astaxanthin fatty acid esters in rainbow trout (*Oncorhynchus mykiss*). In their study, mono-esterified and di-esterified (3S,3′ S)-astaxanthin were purified from the microalga *H. pluvialis* and incorporated into extruded diets and compared with diets containing synthetic racemic astaxanthin (Carophyll Pink) and a total carotenoid extract from the alga. They found that all sources of astaxanthin achieved >4 mg kg^{-1} in the white muscle after 6 weeks feeding, and astaxanthin was deposited in the white muscle in the stereochemical form administered in the diet, i.e., racemic astaxanthin for Carophyll Pink and 100% (3S,3′ S)-astaxanthin for the algal sources. In contrast, epimerization of (3S,3′ S)-astaxanthin from the alga was observed for the astaxanthin esters deposited in the skin of rainbow trout, with a ratio close to 1.0:2.0:1.0 (3S,3′ S:3R,3′ S:3R,3′ R).

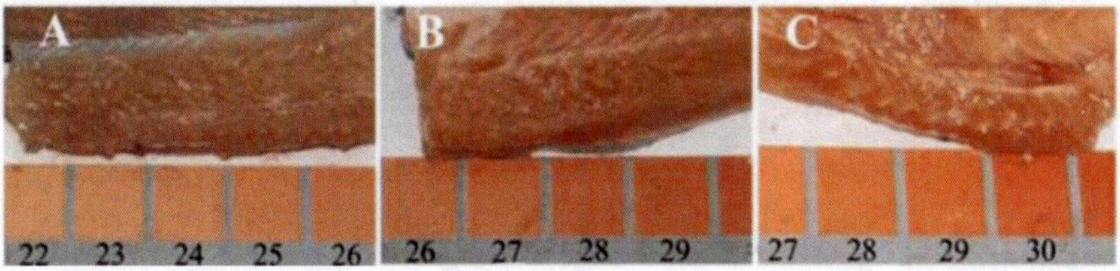

Figure 8. Color of dorsal muscle of *Oncorhynchus mykiss* fed with different diets. Control (A), Sythetic astaxanthin (B) and astaxanthin from *H. pluvialis* (C). (Source: Su F., 2018).

Our recent feeding trials in rainbow trout (*Oncorhynchus mykiss*) suggested that *H. pluvialis* natural astaxanthin was able to replace synthetic astaxanthin as a source of coloring pigment for rainbow trout (Figure 8). The results showed that the color values of rainbow trout muscle were 26 and 27 in the groups of control (Figure 8A) and sythetic astaxanthin (Figure 8B), respectively, while the value was 29 in the group of *H. pluvialis* natural astaxanthin (Figure 8C) (Su F., 2018).

Astaxanthin is used not only in seawater fish but also in freshwater fish. Jagruthi et al., (2014) investigated the effect of astaxanthin at 0, 25, 50, and 100 mg kg^{-1} incorporated in basal feed on immune response and disease resistance in *Cyprinus carpio* against *Aeromonas hydrophila.* Their study suggested that supplementation of astaxanthin at 50 and 100 mg kg^{-1} with the basal diet significantly promoted the growth restores hematology and modulated the immune system in *C. carpio* against *A. hydrophila*.

Sea Urchin

The sea urchin is an economically important species. The gonads of the sea urchins are a highly valued seafood and are considered a prized delicacy in many countries (Ding et al., 2007). The quality of gonad depends on its mass and appearance, especially its color, which is one of the major factors affecting the marketability of sea urchins, and is determined by the composition of carotenoids accumulated in the gonads of sea urchins (Chen et al., 2010). So there were reports about the application of carotenoids- astaxanthin on sea urchin. For example, Peng et al., (2012) reported the effect of the microalgae *H. pluvialis* and *Chorella zofingiensis*, and synthetic astaxanthin on the gonad of the sea urchin *Anthocidaris crassispina*. The basal diet was supplemented with *H. pluvialis*, *C. zofingiensis*, or synthetic astaxanthin, at two levels of astaxanthin (approximately 400 mg kg^{-1} and 100 mg kg^{-1}), to obtain the experimental diets HP1, HP2, CZ1, CZ2, AST1, and AST2, respectively, for two months of feeding experiment. The results showed that the concentrations of astaxanthin in the gonads of the sea urchins fed these experimental diets ranged from 0.15 to 3.01 mg kg^{-1} dry gonad weight. The higher astaxanthin levels (>2.90 mg kg^{-1}) were found in the gonads of the sea urchins fed the diets HP1 (containing 380 mg kg^{-1} of astaxanthins, mostly mono- and diesters) and AST1 (containing 385 mg kg^{-1} of synthetic astaxanthin). The lowest astaxanthin level (0.15 mg kg^{-1}) was detected in the gonads of the sea urchins fed the diet CZ2 (containing 98 mg kg^{-1} of astaxanthins, mostly diesters). Furthermore, the highest canthaxanthin level (7.48 mg kg^{-1}) was found in the gonads of the sea urchins fed the diet CZ1 (containing 387 mg kg^{-1} of astaxanthins and 142 mg kg^{-1} of canthaxanthin), suggesting that astaxanthins, especially astaxanthin esters, might not be assimilated as easily as canthaxanthin by the sea urchins. Their results suggested that sea urchins fed diets containing astaxanthin pigments showed higher incorporation of these known antioxidant constituents, with the resultant seafood products therefore being of potential higher nutritive value.

In summary, the astaxanthin application in aquaculture is currently the major market driver for the pigment and it also plays a key role in enhancing the growth, reproductive performance and immune system in aquaculture animals.

APPLICATION IN HUMAN HEALTH AND NUTRITION

The energy needed by the cell is generated in the mitochondria via multiple oxidative chain reactions, which are accompanied by the production of a large amount of reactive oxygen species (ROS) such as superoxide anion radical ($\cdot O_2^-$), hydrogen peroxide (H_2O_2), hydroxyl radical ($\cdot$ OH), and peroxinitrite anion ($ONOO^-$). These ROS need to be neutralized in order to maintain the proper functions of this cellular component and to protect the cell from degradation and aging (Hussein et al., 2006). Astaxanthin acted as a safeguard against oxidative damage, reacted with ROS much faster than did the protective enzymes (such as superoxide dismutase, peroxidase, catalase and ascorbate peroxidase), and had the strongest antioxidative capacity to protect against lipid peroxidation (Liu et al., 2010) and thus enhanced immune system function and regulated gene expression (Rao et al., 2013). The high anti-oxidant capacity and polar features of astaxanthin make it an amazing nutraceutical for favorable applications in human health and nutrition. A number of articles have been published on the astaxanthin applications in human health and nutrition.

Astaxanthin and Gastric Antral Ulcerations

There are some reports on the cellular effects of astaxanthin. Kim et al., (2005) reported a protective effect of astaxanthin on naproxen-induced and ethanol-induced gastric antral ulcerations in rats in a dose-dependent manner, accompanied by a significant increase in the activities of radicals scavenging enzymes. The randomized double-blind placebo-controlled studies by Kupcinskas et al., (2008) showed different responses of *Helicobacter pylori* negative and positive patients to the treatment of nonulcer dyspepsia with dietary supplements of natural astaxanthin. They concluded that the significantly greater reduction of reflux symptoms was detected in patients treated with the highest dose of the natural astaxanthin and the response was more pronounced in *H. pylori*-infected patients.

Astaxanthin and Cancers

Astaxanthin has the property of anticancer. It has markedly attenuated the promotion of hepatic metastasis induced by restraint stress in mice and this anticancer effect was suggested to be through inhibition of the stress induced lipid peroxidation (Kurihara et al., 2002). Studies on human and animal cells had demonstrated that connexin 43 (Cx43) protein, the most widely expressed connexin in tissues, was up-regulated at the message and protein level by chemopreventive retinoids and astaxanthin, leading to a decreased proliferation and decreased indices of neoplasia. The result showed that combinations of astaxanthin and retinoids were capable of superadditive up-regulation of the tumor suppressor gene connexin 43 (Cx43) and derivatives of astaxanthin induced expression of Cx43 (Hix et al., 2004; Vine et al., 2005), suggesting that astaxanthin has potential anticancer activity.

Astaxanthin and Inflammatory Responses

Astaxanthin could prevent inflammatory processes by blocking the expression of pro-inflammatory genes as a consequence of suppressing the nuclear factor *kappa* B (NF-κB) activation (Lee et al., 2003). It also inhibited the production of nitric oxide (NO) and prostaglandin E2 (PGE2) and the pro-inflammatory cytokines tumor necrosis factor-alpha (TNF-α) and interleukin-1beta (IL-1β). Ohgami et al., (2003) also demonstrated that astaxanthin had the anti-inflammatory effect by suppression of NO, PGE2, and TNF-α production via direct blockage of nitric oxide synthase (NOS) enzyme activity.

Astaxanthin and Nephropathy

Astaxanthin ameliorated the progression and acceleration of diabetic nephropathy in diabetic mice, a rodent model of type 2 diabetes (Naitoa et al., 2003). In our previous study (Liu et al., 2014), the Wistar rats were pre-fed with different doses of astaxanthin-riched *H. pluvialis* powder via orogastric gavage for 30 days. Then, acute kidney injury (AKI) was induced by daily intraperitoneal injection of gentamicin for 7 days. Our result suggested that astaxanthin had the strong preventive effects on AKI in the tested rats.

Astaxanthin and Eye Health

Astaxanthin is beneficial to eye health. The pretreatment of human lens epithelial cells with astaxanthin and xanthophylls lutein and zeaxanthin complex significantly decreased ultraviolet B (UVB) -induced lipid peroxidation and stress signaling (Chitchumroonchokchai et al., 2004). Yamagishi et al., (2014) found that cultures with astaxanthin showed an increase in rat retinal ganglion cells (RGC) viability. They concluded that astaxanthin had a protective effect against RGC death induced by glutamate stress, oxidative stress, and hypoxia, which induced apoptotic and necrotic cell death

Astaxanthin and Skeletal Muscle

The generation of ROS is increased during strenuous exercise as a result of increase in mitochondrial oxygen consumption, leading to lipid peroxidation and skeletal muscle damage. It was found that astaxanthin attenuated exercise-induced damage in mouse skeletal muscle (Aoi et al., 2003) and also attenuated muscular soreness. Furthermore, they investigated the effect of astaxanthin on muscle lipid metabolism in exercise and found that astaxanthin promoted lipid metabolism rather than glucose utilization during exercise via carnitine palmitoyltransferase I (CPT I) activation, which led to improvement of endurance and efficient reduction of adipose tissue with training (Aoi et al., 2008).

Astaxanthin and Skin

Astaxanthin have protective effects on the skin and prevent the photo-aging of the skin. Because the skin is exposed to both endogenous and environmental pro-oxidant agents, leading to ROS generation and possibly damages of DNA, cell membrane lipids, and proteins. The increase of ROS will lead to the modification of the skin antioxidant chemical and enzymatic network and an alteration of cell homeostasis. The *in vitro* research of Lyons et al., (2002), using human skin cell line cultures, had shown that preincubation with an algal extract containing astaxanthin prevented ultraviolet A (UVA)-induced alterations in cellular superoxide dismutase (SOD) activity and cellular glutathione content, and displayed protection against UVA-induced DNA damage. Besides, astaxanthin prevented UV-induced cutaneous inflammation, abnormal keratinization and wrinkling as well as pigmentation of the skin even by its post-irradiation treatment (Imokawa et al., 2018).

Astaxanthin and Erythrocyte

Astaxanthin has the positive influence on an abnormal accumulation of phospholipid hydroperoxides (PLOOH) in the erythrocytes of patients (Kiyotaka et al., 2011). PLOOH were the primary oxidation products of phospholipids and their accumulation in erythrocytes induced a reduction in oxygen transport to the brain, facilitating the progression of dementia (Leijenaar et al., 2017). Kiyotaka et al., (2011) described lower PLOOH levels in the erythrocytes and blood cells of patients treated with astaxanthin with respect to the control (placebo group), demonstrating that this bioactive molecule was responsible for the improvement of erythrocyte antioxidant status.

Astaxanthin and Reproduction

A study based on a self-administered food and supplements frequency questionnaire, had revealed that the higher intake of carotenoids, including astaxanthin, was associated with greater sperm numbers and motility in humans (Eskenazi et al., 2005). The supplementation with astaxanthin improved sperm quality and function in male patients with deficient semen. And it also increased spontaneous or intrauterine insemination-assisted conception rates (Comhaire et al., 2003).

Astaxanthin and Cardiovascular Diseases

Reports have demonstrated a linkage between oxidative stress and the cardiovascular diseases and their consequent implications. The powerful antioxidant astaxanthin can be one of these future candidates (Folsom et al., 1992). Some studies had reported that astaxanthin had myocardial salvage potential of a naturally oriented astaxanthin disuccinate derivative in a rat model of infarction (Gross et al., 2004) and might improve plaque stability in atherosclerosis by decreasing macrophage infiltration, apoptosis, and vulnerability in atheroma of hyperlipidemic rabbits (Hussein et al., 2005a). In preliminary investigations, oral administration of astaxanthin (50 mg kg^{-1} day^{-1}) for 2 weeks induced a significant reduction in blood pressure (BP) in spontaneously hypertensive rats (SHR), but not in the normotensive Wistar Kyoto strain. Another study showed that astaxanthin could further delay the incidence of stroke in the strokeprone SHR-SP upon a 5-week treatment (Hussein et al., 2005a). Zhou et al., (2017) reported that the natural astaxanthin from *H. pluvialis* had also the protective effects on the exercise-induced myocardial injury in rat.

Astaxanthin and Brain

The human Central Nervous System (CNS) included all nerves in the brain and spinal cord and was isolated from the other compartments of the human body through the blood-brain barrier (BBB). The BBB was fundamental to control and restricted the penetration of molecules (e.g., neurotoxins) and cells (e.g., immune cells or infectious agents) from peripheral parts of the body into the CNS. Glia cells of CNS released cytokines, reactive oxygen species (ROS) and reactive nitrogen species (RNS), which could be harmful for neurons and oligodendrocytes when neuroinflammation was not a transient event. There was growing evidence suggesting that a long-standing chronic neuroinflammatory response might lead to neuronal damage, producing neurodegeneration via sustained accumulation of neurotoxic pro-inflammatory mediators (Cho et al., 2018). Besides, an unbalance between ROS production and endogenous mechanisms for detoxification of reactive oxygen intermediates led to neurotoxicity and neurodegeneration. Because astaxanthin could cross the BBB (Petri et al., 2007), it had the potential to treat neurodegenerative diseases.

Attenuating Oxidative Stress in Brain

The CNS was considered highly vulnerable to oxidative stress due to its low cell renewal potential and high cellular metabolism, since this organ required about 25% of total body energy. This energy was fundamental for neuronal connection, axonal transport, and myelination, while mitochondrial activity produced a high amount of ROS. ROS were involved in several signal transduction pathways, such as survival, growth, proliferation and defense mechanisms against microbial infection.

Astaxanthin attenuated oxidative stress induced by amygdala kindling in adult rat hippocampus (Lu et al., 2015; Wen et al., 2015). It alleviated brain aging in rats by attenuating oxidative stress (Wu et al., 2013) and inhibited reactive oxygen species-mediated cellular toxicity in dopaminergic SH-SY5Y cells via mitochondria-targeted protective mechanism (Liu et al., 2009). The anti-oxidant properties of astaxanthin were believed to play an important role in providing protection against inflammation, cancer, aging and macular degeneration related to age in mice (Guerin et al., 2003). Besides, astaxanthin enhanced the activities of antioxidant enzymes in the brain of mice, In the study of Al-Amin et al., (2015), the treatment with astaxanthin significantly ($P < 0.05$) reduced the level of malondialdehyde (MDA), advanced protein oxidation product (APOP), nitric oxide (NO) in the cortex, striatum, hypothalamus, hippocampus and cerebellum in the mice of both young (3 months) and old (16 months) age. Astaxanthin markedly ($P < 0.05$) enhanced the activity of catalase (CAT) and superoxide dismutase (SOD) enzymes while improved the level of glutathione (GSH) in the brain. Overall, improvement of oxidative markers was significantly greater in the young group than the aged animal. They concluded that the activity of astaxanthin was age-dependent, higher in young in compared to the aged brain. Moreover, Mattei et al., (2011) found that the combination of astaxanthin and fish oil enhanced the positive effect on brain health by reducing oxidative stress. In particular, a Wistar rat fed with 1 mg kg^{-1} of astaxanthin and 1 mg kg^{-1} of fish oil presented lipid protection status at the anterior forebrain level. Trolox equivalent antioxidant capacity (TAEC) and Ferric Reducing Antioxidant Power (FRAP) assessed in brain homogenates was found to increase in rats fed with a mix of astaxanthin and fish oil, with respect to only fish oil (Mattei et al., 2011).

Anti-Neuroinflammatory

Some carotenoids had anti-neuroinflammatory effects and with protective properties against oxidative stress in neuronal cell models (Nicholls et al., 2008). Astaxanthin had been shown to have anti-neuroinflammatory. For example, astaxanthin reduced hippocampal and retinal inflammation in streptozotocin-induced diabetic rats, alleviating cognitive deficits, retinal oxidative stress, and depression (Yeh et al., 2016; Zhou et al., 2015; Zhou et al., 2017). The mechanism of action for some carotenoids was the suppression of inflammation pathways through the radical scavenging activity against oxygen-reactive species, but astaxanthin protected neuronal cells from oxidative stress, through the activation of specific pathways, such as Heme oxygenase-1 (HO-1)/NADPH oxidase (NOX) axis and Sp1/NR1 signaling (Ye et al., 2012; Ye et al., 2013).

The anti-neuroinflammatory effects of astaxanthin played an important role in preventing the progression of disorders of the CNS. Astaxanthin blocked the NF-κB-dependent signaling pathway and gene expression of downstream inflammatory mediators like interleukin-1β (IL-1β), interleukin-6 (IL-6) and tumor necrosis factor-α (TNF-α) (Suzuki et al., 2006). Astaxanthin also exhibited its anti-inflammatory actions by inhibiting cyclooxygenase-1 enzyme (COX-1) and nitric oxide (NO) in lipopolysaccharide-stimulated microglial cells (Choi et al., 2008).

Attenuating Cognitive Disorders and Improving Cognitive Functions

Cognitive disorders are a group of mental health diseases that cause several effects on mental abilities, such as learning, problem solving, memory and perception. Recently, it was demonstrated that astaxanthin attenuates cognitive disorders in *in vivo* and *in vitro* models for neurodegenerative diseases (Katagiri et al., 2012; Wu et al., 2015; Che et al., 2018). A study reported that dietary astaxanthin accumulated in the hippocampus and cerebral cortex of rat brains after single and repeated ingestion. And the accumulation of dietary astaxanthin in the cerebral cortex might affect maintenance and improvement of cognitive functions (Manabe et al., 2018). Astaxanthin delayed or ameliorated the cognitive impairment associated with normal aging or alleviated the pathophysiology of various neurodegenerative diseases (Xu et al., 2015; Wen et al., 2015). El-Agamy et al., (2018) investigated the potential effect of astaxanthin as a protective compound able to drastically contrast the decline of cognitive functions induced by doxorubicin (DOX). They concluded that astaxanthin showed neuroprotection and memory-enhancing effects and was able to switch off inflammation and oxidative stress, mitigating the increase of acetylcholinesterase activity and suppressing several pro-apoptotic stimuli.

Improving Learning and Memory

Astaxanthin can improve learning and memory in mice. The impact of astaxanthin-enriched algal (*H.pluvialis*) powder on auxiliary memory improvement was assessed in BALB/c mice pre-supplemented with different dosages of cracked green algal (*H. pluvialis*) powder daily for 30 days. The results of the Morris maze experiment showed that middle dosage of *H. pluvialis* meals (1.3 mg astaxanthin kg^{-1} body weight) significantly shortened the latency and distance required for mice to find a hidden platform (Zhang et al., 2007). The next feeding trial in BALB/c mice for 4 months showed that the natural astaxanthin might improve the memory of middle-aged (9 months) BALB/c mice. Besides, Astaxanthin ameliorated aluminum chloride-induced spatial memory impairment and neuronal oxidative stress in mice (Alamin et al., 2016).

Hussein et al., (2005b) also performed the experiment of Morris water maze in order to study the effects of astaxanthin on the transient ischemia-induced memory impairment in ICR mice. Transient cerebral ischemia was induced by occlusion of carotid arteries. Astaxanthin was given orally to the animals 1 h before occlusion of carotid arteries. Two days after the ischemia, the mice received training trials of 4 trials per day for 5 days, and the time course of change in the latency of escaping to the pool platform was recorded. The swimming time in the platform quadrant was recorded at the probe trial for 1 min after the platform was removed on day 7 of the test. These experiments showed that pretreatment of mice with astaxanthin (55 and 550 mg kg^{-1}) significantly shortened the latency of escaping onto the platform and increased the time of crossing the former platform quadrant in the probe trial (Hussein et al., 2005b). This effect was suggested to be due to the significant antioxidant property of astaxanthin on ischemia-induced free radicals and their consequent pathological cerebral and neural effects. Their studies indicated that astaxanthin might have beneficial effects in preventing the memory deficit in vascular dementia (Hussein et al., 2006).

Others

Astaxanthin has cerebral protection effect. Zhang et al., (2014) found that astaxanthin administration markedly reduced neuronal apoptosis in the early period after subarachnoid hemorrhage (SAH) by modulating the Akt/Bad pathway. Wu et al., (2014) found that the astaxanthin activated nuclear factor erythroid-related factor 2 and the antioxidant responsive element (Nrf2-ARE) pathway in the brain after SAH in Rats and attenuated early brain injury. In the research of Abadie-Guedes et al., (2012), the acute effect of a single Ethanol (EtOH) administration on cortical spreading depression (CSD), which was facilitated by chronic EtOH intake, was investigated in young and adult rats previously (1 hour) treated with astaxanthin. The results showed an antagonistic effect of acute EtOH treatment on CSD propagation that was reverted by astaxanthin. Our feeding trial in APP/PS1 mice (the Alzheimer's Disease-AD model mice) for 4 months suggested that the astaxanthin had beneficial effects on the pathology of AD mice. The study of Lobos et al., (2016) demonstrated the protective effect of astaxanthin on amyloid beta-induced generation of ROS and calcium dysregulation in primary hippocampal neurons.

In summary, astaxanthin, probably due to its strong antioxidant potential, was able to reduce the oxidative stress, progression of neurodegeneration and prevent cognitive dysfunctions, acting on memory and sight.

REFERENCES

Abadie-Guedes, R., Guedes, R. C. A., & Bezerra, R. S. (2012). The impairing effect of acute ethanol on spreading depression is antagonized by astaxanthin in rats of 2 young-adult ages. *Alcoholism: Clinical and Experimental Research, 36*(9).

Al-Amin, M. M., Akhter, S., Hasan, A. T., Alam, T., Nageeb Hasan, S. M., & Saifullah, A. R. et al., (2015). The antioxidant effect of astaxanthin is higher in young mice than aged: a region specific study on brain. *Metabolic Brain Disease, 30*(5), 1237-1246.

Al-Amin, M. M., Reza, H. M., Saadi, H. M., Mahmud, W., Ibrahim, A. A., & Alam, M. M. et al., (2016). Astaxanthin ameliorates aluminum chloride-induced spatial memory impairment and neuronal oxidative stress in mice. *European Journal of Pharmacology,* 777, 60-69.

An, Z., Zhang, Y., & Sun, L. (2018). Effects of dietary astaxanthin supplementation on energy budget and bioaccumulation in *procambarus clarkia* (Girard, 1852) crayfish under microcystin-LR stress. *Toxins, 10*(7), 277.

Aoi, W., Naito, Y., Sakuma, K., Kuchide, M., Tokuda, H., & Maoka, T. et al., (2003). Astaxanthin limits exercise-induced skeletal and cardiac muscle damage in mice. *Antioxidants & Redox Signaling, 5*(1), 139-144.

Aoi, W., Naito, Y., Takanami, Y., Ishii, T., Kawai, Y., & Akagiri, S. et al., (2008). Astaxanthin improves muscle lipid metabolism in exercise via inhibitory effect of oxidative cpt i modification. *Biochemical & Biophysical Research Communications, 366*(4), 0-897.

Arai, S., Mori, T., Miki, W., Yamaguchi, K., Konosu, S., & Satake, M., et al., (1987). Pigmentation of juvenile coho salmon with carotenoid oil extracted from Antarctic krill. *Aquaculture, 66*(3-4), 255-264.

Bjerkeng, B., & Berge, G. M., (2000). Apparent digestibility coefficients and accumulation of astaxanthin e/z isomers in Atlantic salmon (*Salmo salar* L.) and Atlantic halibut (*Hippoglossus hippoglossus* L.). *Comparative Biochemistry and Physiology Part B Biochemistry and Molecular Biology, 127*(3), 0-432.

Bowen, J., Soutar, C., Serwata, R. D., Lagocki, S., White, Daniel., & Davies, Simon. (2002). Utilization of (3s,3′s) - astaxanthin acylesters in pigmentation of rainbow trout (oncorhynchus mykiss). *Aquaculture Nutrition, 8*(1), 59-68.

Capelli, B., Bagchi, D., & Cysewski, G. R., (2013). Synthetic astaxanthin is significantly inferior to algal-based astaxanthin as an antioxidant and may not be suitable as a human nutraceutical supplement. *Nutrafoods, 12*(4), 145-152.

Che H., Li Q., Zhang T., Wang D., Yang L., & Xu J. et al., (2018). Effects of Astaxanthin and Docosahexaenoic-Acid-Acylated Astaxanthin on Alzheimer's Disease in APP/PS1 Double-Transgenic Mice. *Journal of Agricultural and Food Chemistry*, 66,4948-4957.

Chen, G., Xiang, W. Z., Chichung, L., Peng, J., Qiu, J. W., & Feng, C., et al., (2010). A comparative analysis of lipid and carotenoid composition of the gonads of *Anthocidaris crassispina*, *Diadema setosum* and *Salmacis sphaeroides*. *Food Chemistry, 120*(4), 973-977.

Chien, Y. H., & Shiau, W. C., (2005). The effects of dietary supplementation of algae and synthetic astaxanthin on body astaxanthin, survival, growth, and low dissolved oxygen stress resistance of kuruma prawn, *Marsupenaeus japonicus* bate. *Journal of Experimental Marine Biology and Ecology, 318*(2), 201-211.

Chitchumroonchokchai, C., Bomser, J. A., Glamm, J. E., & Failla, M. L. (2004). Xanthophylls and alpha-tocopherol decrease uvb-induced lipid peroxidation and stress signaling in human lens epithelial cells. *Journal of Nutrition, 134*(12), 3225-3232.

Cho, K. S., Shin, M., & Kim, S. (2018). Recent advances in studies on the therapeutic potential of dietary carotenoids in neurodegenerative diseases. *Oxidative Medicine and Cellular Longevity, 2018*(3), 1-13.

Choi, S. K., Park, Y. S., Choi, D. K., & Chang, H. I. (2008). Effects of astaxanthin on the production of no and the expression of cox-2 and inos in lps-stimulated bv2 microglial cells. *J Microbiol Biotechnol, 18*(12), 1990-1996.

Chuchird, N., Rorkwiree, P., & Rairat, T. (2015*). Effect of dietary formic acid and astaxanthin on the survival and growth of pacific white shrimp (Litopenaeus vannamei) and their resistance to vibrio parahaemolyticus*. Springerplus, *4*(1), 1-12.

Comhaire, Frank, H., Mahmoud, & Ahmed. (2003). The role of food supplements in the treatment of the infertile man. *Reproductive Biomedicine Online, 7*(4), 385-391.

Díaz, Ana Cristina, Velurtas, Susana María, Espino, María Laura, & Fenucci, J. L., (2014). Effect of dietary astaxanthin on free radical scavenging capacity and nitrite stress tolerance of postlarvae shrimp, *Pleoticus muelleri. Journal of Agricultural and Food Chemistry, 62*(51), 12326-12331.

Ding, J., Chang, Y., Wang, C., & Cao, X. (2007). Evaluation of the growth and heterosis of hybrids among three commercially important sea urchins in china: *Strongylocentrotus nudus, S. intermedius* and *Anthocidaris crassispina. Aquaculture, 272*(1-4), 0-280.

El-Agamy, S. E., Abdelaziz, A. K., Wahdan, S., Esmat, A., & Azab, S. S. (2018). Astaxanthin ameliorates doxorubicin-induced cognitive impairment (chemobrain) in experimental rat model: impact on oxidative, inflammatory, and apoptotic machineries. *Molecular Neurobiology*, 55(7), 5727-5740.

Eskenazi, B., Kidd, S. A., Marks, A. R., Sloter, E., Block, G., & Wyrobek, A. J. (2005). Antioxidant intake is associated with semen quality in healthy men. *Human Reproduction, 20*(4), 1006.

Folsom, A. R. (1992). Dietary antioxidants and cardiovascular disease. *Annals of the New York Academy of Sciences, 669*(1), 249–258.

Gross, G. J., & Lockwood, S. F. (2004). Cardioprotection and myocardial salvage by a disodium disuccinate astaxanthin derivative (cardax?). *Life Sciences, 75*(2), 0-224.

Guerin, M., Huntley, M. E., & Olaizola, M. (2003). *Haematococcus astaxanthin*: applications for human health and nutrition. *Trends in Biotechnology, 21*(5), 210-216.

Hix, L. M., Lockwood, S. F., & Bertram, J. S. (2004). Upregulation of connexin 43 protein expression and increased gap junctional communication by water soluble disodium disuccinate astaxanthin derivatives. *Cancer Letters, 211*(1), 25-37.

Hussein, G., Goto, H., Oda, S., Iguchi, T., Sankawa, U., & Matsumoto, K. et al., (2005a). Antihypertensive potential and mechanism of action of astaxanthin: ii. vascular reactivity and hemorheology in spontaneously hypertensive rats. *Biological & Pharmaceutical Bulletin, 28*(6), 967.

Hussein, G., Nakamura, M., Zhao, Q., Iguchi, T., Goto, H., & Sankawa, U. et al., (2005b). Antihypertensive and neuroprotective effects of astaxanthin in experimental animals. *Biological & Pharmaceutical Bulletin, 28*(1), 47-52.

Hussein, G., Sankawa, U., Goto, H., Matsumoto, K., & Watanabe, H. (2006). Astaxanthin, a carotenoid with potential in human health and nutrition. *Journal of Natural Products, 69*(3), 443-449.

Imokawa G. (2018). The Xanthophyll Carotenoid Astaxanthin has Distinct Biological Effects to Prevent the Photo-aging of the Skin Even by its Post-irradiation Treatment. *Photochemistry and Photobiology*, doi:10.1111/php.13039.

Jagruthi, C., Yogeshwari, G., Anbazahan, S. M., Mari, L. S., Arockiaraj, J., & Mariappan, P., et al., (2014). Effect of dietary astaxanthin against *Aeromonas hydrophila* infection in common carp, *Cyprinus carpio*. *Fish Shellfish Immunol, 41*(2), 674-680.

Johnston R., Siegfried E., Snell T., Carberry J., Carberry M., & Brown Cody. (2018). Effects of astaxanthin on *Brachionus manjavacas* (Rotifera) population growth. *Aquaculture Research*, 49, 2278–2287.

Ju, Z. Y., Deng, D. F., & Dominy, W., (2012). A defatted microalgae (*Haematococcus pluvialis*) meal as a protein ingredient to partially replace fishmeal in diets of pacific white shrimp (*Litopenaeus vannamei*, boone, 1931). *Aquaculture, 354-355*(none).

Katagiri, M., Satoh, A., Tsuji, S., & Shirasawa, T. (2012). Effects of astaxanthin-rich *haematococcus pluvialis* extract on cognitive function: a randomised, double-blind, placebo-controlled study. *Journal of Clinical Biochemistry and Nutrition, 51*(2), 102-107.

Kim, J. H., Choi, S. K., Choi, S. Y., Kim, H. K., & Chang, H. I. (2005). Suppressive effect of astaxanthin isolated from the xanthophyllomyces dendrorhous mutant on ethanol-induced gastric mucosal injury in rats. *Journal of the Agricultural Chemical Society of Japan, 69*(7), 6.

Kiyotaka, N., Takehiro, K., Taiki, M., Gregor, C. B., Fumiko, K., & Akira, S. et al., (2011). Antioxidant effect of astaxanthin on phospholipid peroxidation in human erythrocytes. *British Journal of Nutrition, 105*(11), 9.

Kupcinskas, L., Lafolie, P., Åke Lignell, Kiudelis, G., Jonaitis, L., & Adamonis, K., et al., (2008). Efficacy of the natural antioxidant astaxanthin in the treatment of functional dyspepsia in patients with or withouwithout the licobacter pyloriinfection: a prospective, randomized, double blind, and placebo-controlled study. *Phytomedicine, 15*(6), 391-399.

Kurihara, H., Koda, H., Asami, S., Kiso, Y., & Tanaka, T. (2002). Contribution of the antioxidative property of astaxanthin to its protective effect on the promotion of cancer metastasis in mice treated with restraint stress. *Life Sciences, 70*(21), 2509-2520.

Lee, S. J., Bai, S. K., Lee, K. S., Namkoong, S., Na, H. J., & Ha, K. S. et al., (2003). Astaxanthin inhibits nitric oxide production and inflammatory gene expression by suppressing I(kappa)B kinase-dependent NF-kappaB activation. *Molecules & Cells, 16*(1), 97-105.

Leijenaar, J. F., Maurik, I. S. V., Kuijer, J. P. A., Flier, W. M. V. D., Scheltens, P., & Barkhof, F. et al., (2017). Lower cerebral blood flow in subjects with alzheimer'sAlzheimer's dementia, mild cognitive impairment, and subjective cognitive decline using 2d phase-contrast mriMRI. *Alzheimers & Dementia Diagnosis Assessment & Disease Monitoring, 9*, 76-83.

Li Hu and Liu Jianguo (2019), Effects of defatted *Haematococcus pluvialis* meal (DHPM) supplementation on the growth performance, and the carotenoid content and composition in the rotifer (*Brachionus plicatilis*). *Aquaculture*, https://doi.org/10.1016/ j.aquaculture.2019. 02.027

Liu J. G., Zhang X. L., Sun Y. H., Lin W. (2010). Antioxidative capacity and enzyme activity in *haematococcus pluvialis* cells exposed to superoxide free radicals. *Chinese Journal of Oceanology and Limnology, 28*(1), 1-9.

Liu Xiaohui, Wang Baojie, Li Yongfu, Wang Lei, Liu Jianguo (2018). Effects of dietary botanical and synthetic astaxanthin on E/Z and R/S isomer composition, growth performance, and antioxidant capacity of white shrimp, *Litopenaeus vannamei*, in the nursery phase. *Invertebrate Survival Journal*, 15, 131-140.

Liu, J. G., He, J., Zhang, Y., Gao, H., Liu, D. Y., & Pang, T. (2014). Effects of Microalgal Carotenoids on Acute Renal Injury Prophylaxis in Male Wistar Rats. *National conference on Marine biotechnology and innovative medicine*, Chifeng, China, 2014.08.

Liu, X., Shibata, T., Hisaka, S., & Osawa, T. (2009). Astaxanthin inhibits reactive oxygen species-mediated cellular toxicity in dopaminergic sh-sy5y cells via mitochondria-targeted protective mechanism. *Brain Research, 1254*, 18-27.

Lobos P., Bruna B., Cordova A., Barattini P., Galáz JL., & Adasme T., et al., (2016). Astaxanthin Protects Primary Hippocampal Neurons against Noxious Effects of Aβ-Oligomers. *Neural Plasticity*, 2016.

Long Xiaowen, Wu Xugan, Zhao Lei, Liu Jianguo, Cheng Yongxu (2017). Effects of dietary supplementation with *Haematococcus pluvialis*, cell powder on coloration, ovarian development and antioxidation capacity of adult female Chinese mitten crab, *Eriocheir sinensis*. *Aquaculture*, 473, 545-553.

Lu, Y., Xie, T., He, X. X., Mao, Z. F., Jia, L. J., & Wang, W. P. et al., (2015). Astaxanthin rescues neuron loss and attenuates oxidative stress induced by amygdala kindling in adult rat hippocampus. *Neuroscience Letters, 597*, 49-53.

Lyons, N. M., & O'Brien, N. M. (2002). Modulatory effects of an algal extract containing astaxanthin on uva-irradiated cells in culture. *Journal of Dermatological Science, 30*(1), 73-84.

Manabe, Y., Komatsu, T., Seki, S., & Sugawara, T. (2018). Dietary astaxanthin can accumulate in the brain of rats. *Bioscience, Biotechnology, and Biochemistry*, 1-4.

Mattei, R., Polotow, T. G., Vardaris, C. V., Guerra, B. A., José Roberto Leite, & Otton, R. et al., (2011). Astaxanthin limits fish oil-related oxidative insult in the anterior forebrain of wistar rats: putative anxiolytic effects? *Pharmacology Biochemistry & Behavior, 99*(3), 349-355.

Naitoa, Y., Uchiyama, K., Aoi, W., Hasegawa, G., Nakamura, N., & Yoshida, N. et al., (2013). Prevention of diabetic nephropathy by treatment with astaxanthin in diabetic db/db mice. *BioFactors, 39*(5), 590-590.

Nicholls, D. G. (2008). Oxidative stress and energy crises in neuronal dysfunction. *Annals of the New York Academy of Sciences, 1147*(1), 53-60.

Niu, J., Li, C. H., Liu, Y. J., Tian, L. X., Chen, X., & Huang, Z. et al., (2012). Dietary values of astaxanthin and canthaxanthin in penaeus monodon in the presence and absence of cholesterol supplementation: effect on growth, nutrient digestibility and tissue carotenoid composition. *British Journal of Nutrition, 108*(01), 80-91.

Ohgami, K., Shiratori, K., Kotake, S., Nishida, T., Mizuki, N., & Yazawa, K. et al., (2003). Effects of astaxanthin on lipopolysaccharide-induced inflammation *in vitro* and *in vivo*. *Investigative Opthalmology & Visual Science, 44*(6), 2694.

Peng, J., Yuan, J. P., & Wang, J. H. (2012). Effect of diets supplemented with different sources of astaxanthin on the gonad of the sea urchin *Anthocidaris crassispina*. *Nutrients, 4*(8), 922-934.

Petri, D., & Lundebye, A. K. (2007). Tissue distribution of astaxanthin in rats following exposure to graded levels in the feed. *Comparative*

Biochemistry and Physiology Part C Toxicology & Pharmacology, 145(2), 202-209.

Rao, A. R., Sindhuja, H. N., Dharmesh, S. M., Sankar, K. U., Sarada, R., & Ravishankar, G. A. (2013). Effective inhibition of skin cancer, tyrosinase, and antioxidative properties by astaxanthin and astaxanthin esters from the green alga *haematococcus pluvialis. Journal of Agricultural & Food Chemistry, 61*(16), 3842-3851.

Su Fang (2018). *A study on the structure distribution of carotenoids in algae, shrimps, crabs and fishes and the isomerization of astaxanthin.* A Dissertation Submitted to University of Chinese Academy of Sciences, 95-97.

Suzuki, Y., Ohgami, K., Shiratori, K., Jin, X. H., Ilieva, I., & Koyama, Y. et al., (2006). Suppressive effects of astaxanthin against rat endotoxin-induced uveitis by inhibiting the nf-κb signaling pathway. *Experimental Eye Research, 82*(2), 0-281.

Vine, A. L., Leung, Y. M., & Bertram, J. S. (2005). Transcriptional regulation of connexin 43 expression by retinoids and carotenoids: similarities and differences. *Molecular Carcinogenesis, 43*(2), 75-85.

Wen, X., Huang, A., Hu, J., Zhong, Z., Liu, Y., & Li, Z., et al., (2015). Neuroprotective effect of astaxanthin against glutamate-induced cytotoxicity in ht22 cells: involvement of the akt/gsk-3β pathway. *Neuroscience, 303*, 558-568.

Wu Xugan, Zhao Lei, Long Xiaowen, Liu Jianguo, Su Fang, Cheng Yongxu (2017). Effects of dietary supplementation of *Haematococcus pluvialis* powder on gonadal development, coloration and antioxidant capacity of adult male Chinese mitten crab (*Eriocheir Sinensis*). *Aquaculture Research,* 48, 1-10.

Wu, H., Niu, H., Shao, A., Wu, C., Dixon, B. J., & Zhang, J. et al., (2015). Astaxanthin as a potential neuroprotective agent for neurological diseases. *Marine Drugs, 13*(9), 5750-5766.

Wu, Q., Zhang, X. S., Wang, H. D., Zhang, X., Yu, Q., & Li, W. et al., (2014). Astaxanthin activates nuclear factor erythroid-related, factor 2 and the antioxidant responsive element (nrf2-are) pathway in the brain after subarachnoid hemorrhage in rats and attenuates early brain injury. *Marine Drugs, 12*(12), 6125.

Wu, W., Wang, X., Xiang, Q., Meng, X., Peng, Y., & Du, N., et al., (2013). Astaxanthin alleviates brain aging in rats by attenuating oxidative stress and increasing bdnf levels. *Food & Function, 5*(1), 158-166.

Xie S. W., Fang W. P., Wei D., Liu Y. J., Yin P., & Niu J., et al., (2018). Dietary supplementation of, *Haematococcus pluvialis*, improved the immune capacity and low salinity tolerance ability of post-larval white shrimp, *Litopenaeus vannamei*. *Fish & Shellfish Immunology, 80*, 452-457.

Xu, L., Zhu, J., Yin, W., & Ding, X. (2015). Astaxanthin improves cognitive deficits from oxidative stress, nitric oxide synthase and inflammation through upregulation of pi3k/akt in diabetes rat. *International Journal of Clinical & Experimental Pathology, 8*(6), 6083-6094.

Yamagishi, R., & Aihara, M. (2014). Neuroprotective effect of astaxanthin against rat retinal ganglion cell death under various stresses that induce apoptosis and necrosis. *Molecular Vision, 20*(2), 1796-1805.

Ye, Q., Huang, B., Zhang, X. D., Zhu, Y., & Chen, X. (2012). Astaxanthin protects against mpp(+)-induced oxidative stress in pc12 cells via the ho-1/nox2 axis. *BMC Neuroscience, 13*(1), 156-156.

Ye, Q., Zhang, X., Huang, B., Zhu, Y., & Chen, X. (2013). Astaxanthin suppresses mpp+-induced oxidative damage in pc12 cells through a sp1/nr1 signaling pathway. *Marine Drugs, 11*(4), 1019-1034.

Yeh, P. T., Huang, H. W., Yang, C. M., Yang, W. S., & Yang, C. H. (2016). Astaxanthin inhibits expression of retinal oxidative stress and inflammatory mediators in streptozotocin-induced diabetic rats. *PLOS ONE, 11*.

Ytres tøyl, T., & Bjerkeng, B. (2007). Intraperitoneal and dietary administration of astaxanthin in rainbow trout (*Oncorhynchus mykiss*) — plasma uptake and tissue distribution of geometrical e/z isomers. *Comparative Biochemistry & Physiology Part B Biochemistry & Molecular Biology, 147*(2), 0-259.

Zhang Xiaoli, Pan Lishan, Wei Xiaoli, Gao Hong, Liu Jianguo (2007). Impact of astaxanthin-enriched algal powder of *Haematococcus pluvialison* memory improvement in BALB/c mice. *Environmental Geochemistry & Health*, 29(6), 483-489.

Zhang, C. S., Su, F., Li, S. H., Yu, Y., Xiang, J. H., & Liu, J. G., et al., (2018). Isolation and identification of the main carotenoid pigment from a new variety of the ridgetail white prawn, *exopalaemon carinicauda. Food Chemistry*, S0308814618311282-.

Zhang, X. S., Zhang, X., Wu, Q., Li, W., Zhang, Q. R., & Wang, C. X. et al., (2014). Astaxanthin alleviates early brain injury following subarachnoid hemorrhage in rats: possible involvement of akt/bad signaling. *Marine Drugs, 12*(8), 4291.

Zhou H. T., Cao J. M., Gong P., Niu Y. L., Wang C., & Wang Biao. (2017). The protective effects of *haematococcus Haematococcus pluvialis* on the exercise-induced myocardial injury in rat. *Chinese Journal of Applied Physiology, 33*(6), 539.

Zhou, X. Y., Zhang, F., Hu, X. T., Chen, J., Tang, R. X., & Zheng, K. Y. et al., (2017). Depression can be prevented by astaxanthin through inhibition of hippocampal inflammation in diabetic mice. *Brain Research, 1657*, 262-268.

Zhou, X., Zhang, F., Hu, X., Chen, J., Wen, X., & Sun, Y. et al., (2015). Inhibition of inflammation by astaxanthin alleviates cognition deficits in diabetic mice. *Physiology & Behavior*, 151,412-420.

In: An Essential Guide to Astaxanthin ISBN: 978-1-53615-571-6
Editor: Paul A. Melborne

Chapter 2

ASTAXANTHIN BIOSYNTHESIS IN *HAEMATOCOCCUS PLUVIALIS*: METABOLIC PROCESS, FUNCTION, AND BIOTECHNOLOGICAL APPLICATIONS

Litao Zhang[1,2,3], Chunhui Zhang[1,2], Ran Xu[1,2] and Jianguo Liu[1,2,3,*]

[1]CAS Key Laboratory of Experimental Marine Biology, Center for Ocean Mega-Science, Institute of Oceanology, Chinese Academy of Sciences, Qingdao, China

[2]Laboratory for Marine Biology and Biotechnology, Qingdao National Laboratory for Marine Science and Technology, Aoshanwei Town, Jimo, Qingdao, China

[3]National-Local Joint Engineering Research Center for *Haematococcus pluvialis* and Astaxanthin Products, Yunnan Alphy Biotech Co., Ltd., Chuxiong, China

[*] Corresponding Author's E-mail: jgliu@qdio.ac.cn.

ABSTRACT

Astaxanthin has important applications in the nutraceutical, cosmetic, food and feed industries due to its extraordinary antioxidant capability. Unicellular green alga *Haematococcus pluvialis* is recognized as one of the most promising producer of astaxanthin in nature due to its exceptional ability to accumulate large amounts of astaxanthin under environmental stresses. In this review, the terms and concepts of the cell forms of *H. pluvialis* at various cell cycles stages are re-defined in an effort to avoid confusion and awkward phrasing. The changes of pigments (including chlorophyll and carotenoids) and astaxanthin geometrical isomers are elucidated during the incubation in *H. pluvialis* under environmental stresses. Changes in photosynthetic behaviors and photoprotective mechanisms during astaxanthin accumulation are clarified. The astaxanthin metabolic process and regulation are elucidated through analyzing the relationship between astaxanthin biosynthesis and chlororespiration, photorespiration, fatty acid biosynthesis. Meanwhile, an unknown bioactive substance by *H. pluvialis*, which can feed back influence cell growth and transformation from motile cells into non-motile cells, has been revealed. Cultivation of *H. pluvialis* for astaxanthin production in phototrophic, heterotrophic, mixotrophic and heterotrophic-phototrophic culture modes are presented. The biological contamination control during cultivation of *H. pluvialis* is analyzed. In the near future, the genome sequencing and genetic toolbox development will affect significantly future advancement in *H. pluvialis* and astaxanthin biosynthesis research. Mass cultivation of *H. pluvialis* is already physically and economically feasible and profitable, and this industry is bound to expand.

INTRODUCTION

Astaxanthin (3,3'-dihydroxy-β,β-carotene-4,4'-dione) is commonly used not only as a pigmentation source in aquaculture and the poultry industries (Sommer et al. 1991; Benemann 1992), but also has potential clinical applications due to its powerful antioxidant properties, which is higher than that of β-carotene and α-tocopherol (Guerin et al. 2003; Goswami et al. 2010; Liu et al. 2016). Astaxanthin can be produced in various amounts by a number of microalgae, such as *Chlorella zofingiensis*, *Haematococcus pluvialis*, *Chlamydocapsa* spp.,

Chlamydomonas nivalis, *Chloromonas nivalis*, *Neochloris wimmeri*, *Protosiphon botryoides*, *Scenedesmus* sp., *Scotiellopsis oocystiformis* (Orosa et al. 2000; Remias et al. 2005; Leya et al. 2009; Han et al. 2013). Of these species, *H. pluvialis*, a unicellular green alga, is recognized as one of the most promising producers of astaxanthin in nature due to its exceptional ability to accumulate large amounts of astaxanthin under unfavorable conditions (Boussiba 2000; Han et al. 2013; Wang et al. 2013; Chen et al. 2015; Giannelli et al. 2015). Under stress conditions, such as high light, high salinity, and nutrient deprivation, *H. pluvialis* cells start to increase their volume drastically, transform from green motile vegetative cells with flagella to red, non-motile, mature cysts (Boussiba and Vonshak 1991; Kobayashi 2003), full of astaxanthin with no intermediates of the astaxanthin biosynthetic pathway remaining (Boussiba et al. 1999). The biosynthesis of astaxanthin is usually accompanied by the changes of physiological and molecular characteristics in *H. pluvialis*.

To produce astaxanthin using *H. pluvialis*, a two-step with three-phase culture protocol was developed (Wang et al. 2013; Liu et al. 2016; Zhang et al. 2017b). In the first step, favorable growth conditions are provided to accelerate *H. pluvialis* cell growth and to obtain a high biomass (cell growth phase); in the second step, stress conditions are provided to induce cell transformation from green motile cells to non-motile cells (cell transformation phase), and to induce the accumulation of astaxanthin (astaxanthin accumulation phase). However, large-scale, mass cultivation of *H. pluvialis* to obtain optimal astaxanthin production is very challenging because cell growth and astaxanthin accumulation are affected by many interactive factors.

To help in optimizing astaxanthin production, in this review, the changes of pigments (including chlorophyll and carotenoids) and astaxanthin geometrical isomers were elucidated during the incubation in *H. pluvialis* under environmental stresses. Changes in photosynthetic behaviors and photoprotective mechanisms during astaxanthin accumulation were clarified. The astaxanthin metabolic process and regulation were elucidated through analyzing the relationship between astaxanthin biosynthesis and photosynthesis, chlororespiration, photorespiration, and fatty acid biosynthesis. Cultivation of *H. pluvialis* for astaxanthin production in phototrophic, heterotrophic, mixotrophic and heterotrophic-phototrophic culture modes are presented. The biological contamination control during cultivation of *H. pluvialis* is analyzed. The genome sequencing and genetic toolbox development will affect significantly future advancement in *H. pluvialis* and astaxanthin biosynthesis research.

LIFE HISTORY OF *H. PLUVIALIS*

The reproduction of *H. pluvialis* is complex, having several cell types and cell cycles (Elliot 1934; Liu et al. 2016; Zhang et al. 2017a). The complicated life history of *H. pluvialis* can be divided into two stages: the motile stage and the non-motile stage (Han et al. 2013; Liu et al. 2016; Zhang et al. 2017a). All the cells can be classified into forms as follows: motile cell, non-motile cell, zoospore, and aplanospore. However, many terms such as zoospore, flagellated cell, motile cell, red cell, green cell, palmella, non-motile cell, aplanospore, and akinete have appeared in many articles and may result in confusion. Some of these terms are misused. Therefore, Zhang et al. (2017a) re-defined the terms and concepts of the cell forms of *H. pluvialis* at various cell cycles stages (Figure 1).

The main cell proliferation, both in the motile phase and non-motile phase in *H. pluvialis*, is by asexual reproduction (Figure 2). Under normal growth conditions, a motile cell usually produces two, sometimes four, and exceptionally eight zoospores. Under unfavorable conditions, the motile cell loses its flagella and transforms into a non-motile cell, and the non-motile cell usually produces 2, 4 or 8 aplanospores, and occasionally 20-32 aplanospores, which further develop into non-motile cells. Under suitable conditions, the non-motile cell is also able to release zoospores. The larger non-motile cells produce more than 16 zoospores, and the smaller ones produce 4 or 8 zoospores. Vegetative reproduction is by direct cell division in the motile phase and by occasional cell budding in the non-motile phase.

There is, as yet, no convincing direct evidence for sexual reproduction (Liu et al. 2016; Zhang et al. 2017a).

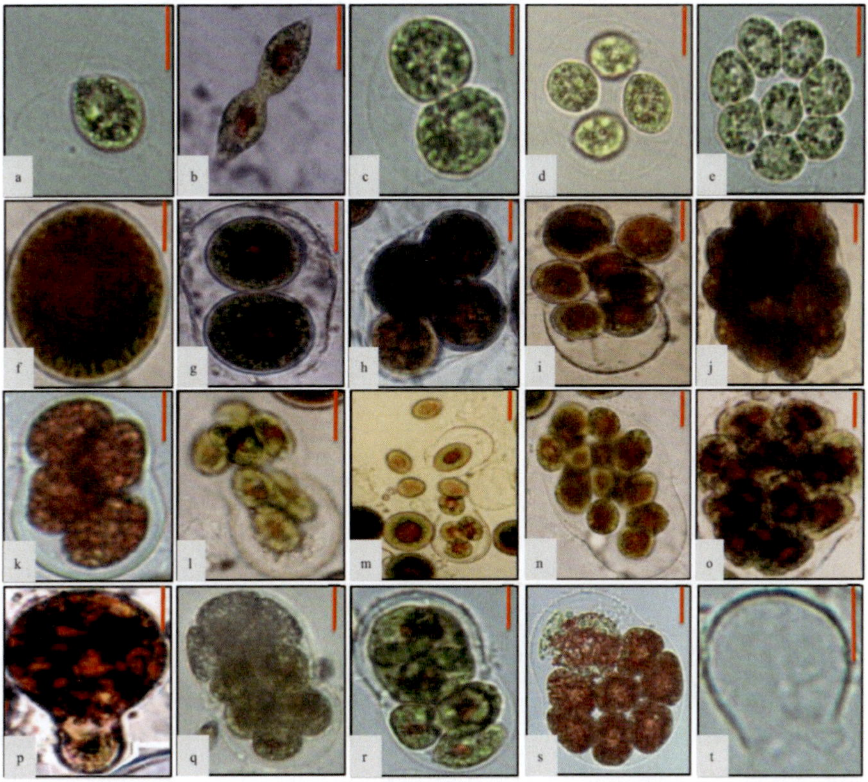

Figure 1. The cell forms of *Haematococcus pluvialis* (Zhang et al. 2017a).
a. motile cell; b. vegetative reproduction by direct cell division in the motile phase; c. sporangium with two zoospores; d. sporangium with four zoospores; e. sporangium with eight zoospores; f. non-motile cell; g. sporangium with two aplanospores; h. sporangium with four aplanospores; i. sporangium with eight aplanospores being released; j. sporangium with >20 aplanospores; k. sporangium with 4 zoospores; l. sporangium with 8 zoospores being released; m. the moment of zoospores release; n. sporangium with 16 zoospores; o. sporangium with >20 zoospores; p. vegetative reproduction by cell budding in the nonmotile phase; q–r. unsynchronized cell division in sporangia during the process of zoospores formation; s. autolysis of some zoospores within the sporangium; t. theca after spores release. The length of each bar represents 10 μm.

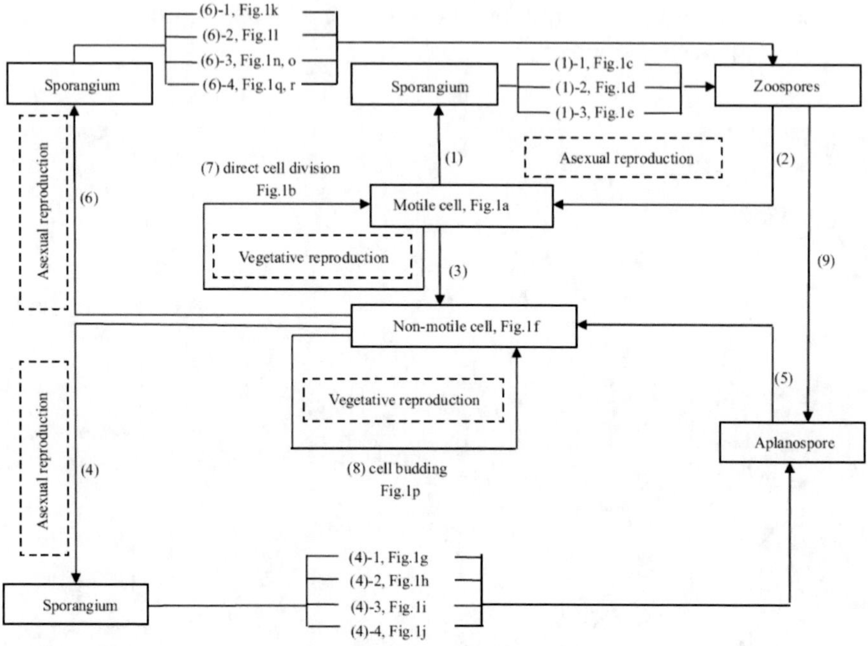

Figure 2. Proliferation patterns and cell cycles in *Haematococcus pluvialis* (Zhang et al. 2017a).

Under normal growth conditions, the motile cells usually produce two (1-1), sometimes four (1-2), and exceptionally eight (1-3) zoospores by asexual reproduction through formation of sporangia (1), and released zoospores are then transformed into motile cells (2). Under unfavorable conditions, motile cells lose their flagella and transform into non-motile cells directly (3), and the non-motile cells usually produce 2 (4-1), 4 (4-2) or 8 aplanospores (4-3), and occasionally 20-32 aplanospores (4-4) through formation of sporangia (4) by asexual reproduction, and further develop into non-motile cells (5). Under suitable conditions, non-motile cells are also able to release zoospores through formation of sporangia (6), in which the bigger non-motile cell produces more than 16 zoospores (6-3), and the smaller one produces 8 (6-2) or 4 zoospores (6-1), occasionally with unsynchronized cell division in some sporangia (6-4). Vegetative reproduction occasionally happens by direct cell division in the motile stage (7) and by cell budding in the non-motile stage (8). (9) Under stressed conditions, zoospores transform into aplanospores in sporangia or undergo autolysis.

PHYSIOLOGICAL AND BIOCHEMICAL CHARACTERISTICS DURING ASTAXANTHIN ACCUMULATION

Pigments

During astaxanthin accumulation in *H. pluvialis*, the chlorophyll level decreased (Zhang et al. 2016a). As for astaxanthin quality, a low content of chlorophyll is an indicator of high quality astaxanthin produced by outdoor mass-scale cultivation, because pheophorbide resulting from degradation of chlorophyll is an allergen (Tsuchiya et al. 1999; Guang 2008). The precursors of astaxanthin synthesis are the so-called 'primary' carotenoids (lycopene, carotene, lutein, zeaxanthin, canthaxanthin and echinenone), which are related to astaxanthin biosynthesis in *H. pluvialis* (Harker et al. 1996; Lemoine and Schoefs 2010). Lutein and zeaxanthin, which can act through the xanthophyll cycle and interconvert, are the most abundant precursors in *H. pluvialis* (Harker et al. 1996). The relative content of lutein and zeaxanthin decreased during astaxanthin accumulation (Figure 2), leading to inhibition of xanthophyll cycle.

The stereochemistry of astaxanthin includes the chiral and geometric isomers mainly (Bernhard 1989). The geometrical isomers compositions were more complex: most of astaxanthin are all-trans-astaxanthin, a small amount of astaxanthin is cis-astaxanthin, including 9-cis-astaxanthin, 13-cis-astaxanthin and little 15-cis-astaxanthin (Yang 2015). Many studies have shown that the cis- and trans-astaxanthin have significant differences in stability and in antioxidant scavenging activity, e.g., against the DPPH radical, ABTS radical and super-oxide anion (Liu et al. 2007). The proportion of astaxanthin geometrical isomers was fluctuating during astaxanthin accumulation in *H. pulvialis* (Figure 3). The proportion of all-trans-astaxanthin increased firstly and then decreased. The proportion of

13-cis-astaxanthin decreased gradually during astaxanthin accumulation phase. The proportion of 9-cis-astaxanthin was stable. Many studies have shown that all-*trans*-isomers can convert to *cis*-isomers by isomerization (Doering et al. 1995; Gao et al. 1996). The specific mechanism leading to astaxanthin isomerization in *H. pulvialis* needs further studies.

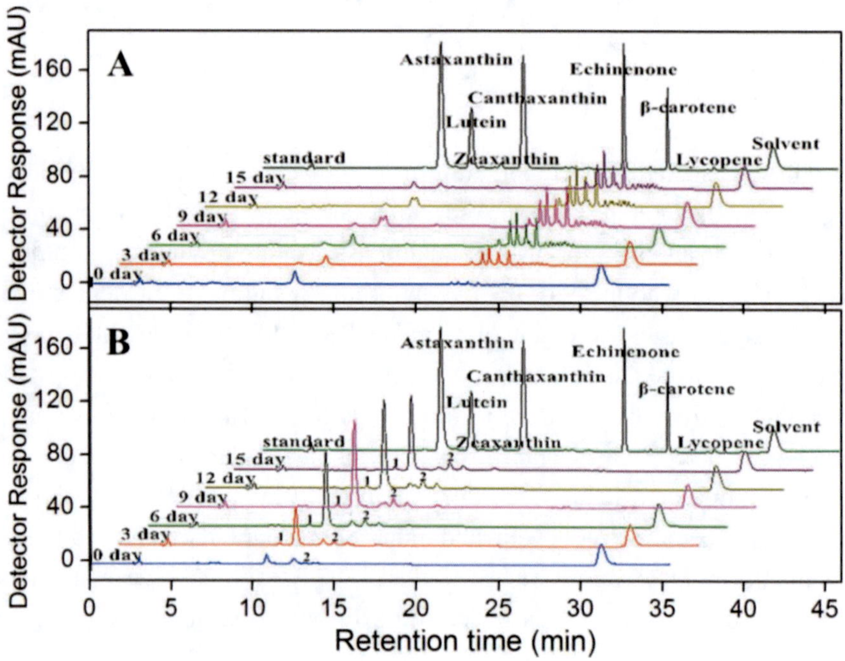

Figure 3. HPLC chromatogram of extracts of *H. pluvialis* during outdoor incubation, without enzymatic hydrolysis (A), after enzymatic hydrolysis (B).
Peaks 1 and 2 are 13-cis-astaxanthin and 9-cis-astaxanthin, respectively.

Photosynthetic Behaviors

The corresponding difference kinetics between cells incubated for 3, 5, 7 or 9 d and cells incubated for 1 d ($\Delta W = W - W_{(\text{cells incubated for 1 d})}$) are also depicted. The difference kinetics ΔW_{OJ} and ΔW_{OK} reveal the K-band (at about 300 μs) and L-band (at about 150 μs) respectively. The chlorophyll *a* fluorescence transient is possible to calculate several phenomenological and biophysical expressions of photosynthetic behaviors. The enhanced J-step indicates increased the over-reduction of PSII acceptor sides. The higher L-band indicates a lower energetic connectivity of the PSII units, which results in a poorer utilization of the excitation energy and a lower stability of the system. The enhanced K-band indicates increased damaged to the donor side of PSII. The maximal amplitude of fluorescence in the I-P phase of the OJIP transient reflects the pool size of end electron acceptors.

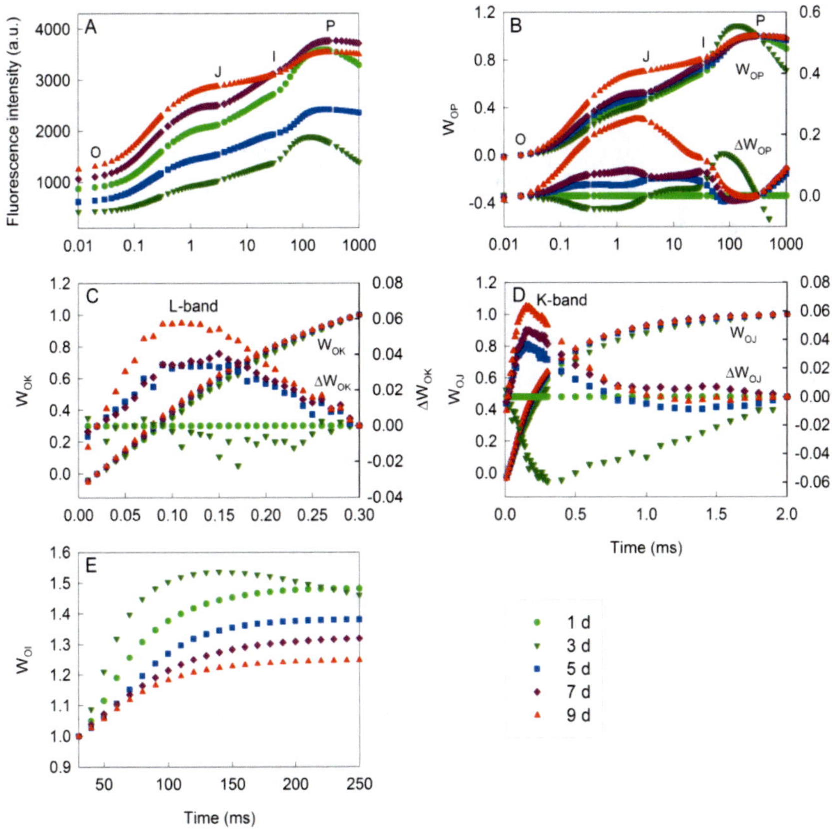

Figure 4. The chlorophyll *a* fluorescence (OJIP) transients during cell transformation and astaxanthin accumulation in *H. pluvialis* (A). The normalization of fluorescence transients between the OP (B), OK (C), OJ (D) and OI (E) phases (Zhang et al. 2017b).

Stress conditions will induce *H. pulvialis* cell transformation from green motile cells to non-motile cells (cell transformation phase), and to induce the accumulation of astaxanthin (astaxanthin accumulation phase). During cell transformation, the light absorption and photosynthetic electron transport became much more efficient, the photosynthetic capacity increased (Figure 4; Zhang et al. 2017b).

During astaxanthin accumulation, the photosystem (PS) I and PSII acceptor sides were over-reduction, the PSII units were less grouped, the donor side of PSII was impaired. It suggests the capacity and efficiency of photosynthetic energy utilization decreased significantly, the balance between photosynthetic light absorption and energy utilization was disturbed (Figure 4; Zhang et al. 2017b). In addition, the imbalance between light absorption and utilization will cause the over-excitation of PSII reaction centers during astaxanthin accumulation in *H. pulvialis* (Zhang et al. 2011).

The astaxanthin accumulation is strongly light-induced processes for *H. pluvialis* (Kobayashi et al. 1992; Steinbrenner and Linden 2000; 2003). However, under high light condition, there are two major sites of reactive oxygen species (ROS) generation in chloroplasts: the end of photosynthetic electron transport chain (acceptor side of PSI) and the PSII reaction centers (Zhang et al. 2011; 2017b; Mittler 2002). The over-reduction of the PSI acceptor side and the over-excitation of PSII reaction centers during astaxanthin accumulation in *H. pluvialis* would inevitably enhance the generation of ROS, leading to more severe photoinhibition (or photodamage) under high light. *H. pluvialis* cells need to induce defence mechanisms to prevent the generation of ROS during astaxanthin accumulation.

Photoprotection

Excess light energy will accelerate the generation of reactive oxygen species (ROS), leading to photoinhibition (Zhang et al. 2011; 2017b). In order to escape from exposure to excess light, most plants have evolved various defence mechanisms to prevent the generation of ROS, such as non-photochemical quenching (NPQ), PSI cyclic electron transport (CEF-PSI) and antioxidant enzymes (Niyogi 2000; Mittler 2002; Zhang et al. 2017b). During astaxanthin accumulation in *H. pluvialis*, the NPQ and antioxidant enzymes capacities decreased and CEF-I activity did not change, but NPQ, CEF-I and antioxidant enzyme activities are extremely higher over time. The NPQ, CEF-I and antioxidant enzymes might play an important role in photoprotection of *H. pluvialis* cells during astaxanthin accumulation. Astaxanthin can also protect *H. pluvialis* cells against oxidative stress (Kobayashi 2000). In the previous study, the role of two distinct antioxidative mechanisms, the defensive enzyme system and the astaxanthin, were compared in *H. pluvialis* (Liu et al. 2010). As an antioxidant, astaxanthin is more efficient than the defensive enzyme system.

Under photoinhibitory conditions, the level of photoinhibition (or photodamage) decreased significantly over time during astaxanthin accumulation, although the PSI acceptor side was over-reduction and the PSII reaction centers were over-excitation during astaxanthin accumulation in *H. pluvialis* (Zhang et al. 2017b). It concludes NPQ, PTOX, CEF-I, defensive enzymes (SOD, APX and CAT) and the accumulation of amounts of astaxanthin can protect *H. pluvialis* cells against photoinhibition (or photodamage) during astaxanthin accumulation.

Metabolic Changes Using Comparative Transcriptome Analysis

To approach a fuller understanding of the complex metabolic changes, especially astaxanthin biosynthesis, occurring during transformation of green to intermediate cells and the formation of non-motile resting cells, a comparative transcriptome study was conducted during cell transformation and astaxanthin accumulation in *H. pluvialis* (Li et al. 2018). During cell transformation and astaxanthin accumulation, seven specified developmental points with perceptible color difference were sampled and sequenced using an Illumina NextSeq500 Sequencer. After pairwise comparison, 2,674 DEGs were identified.

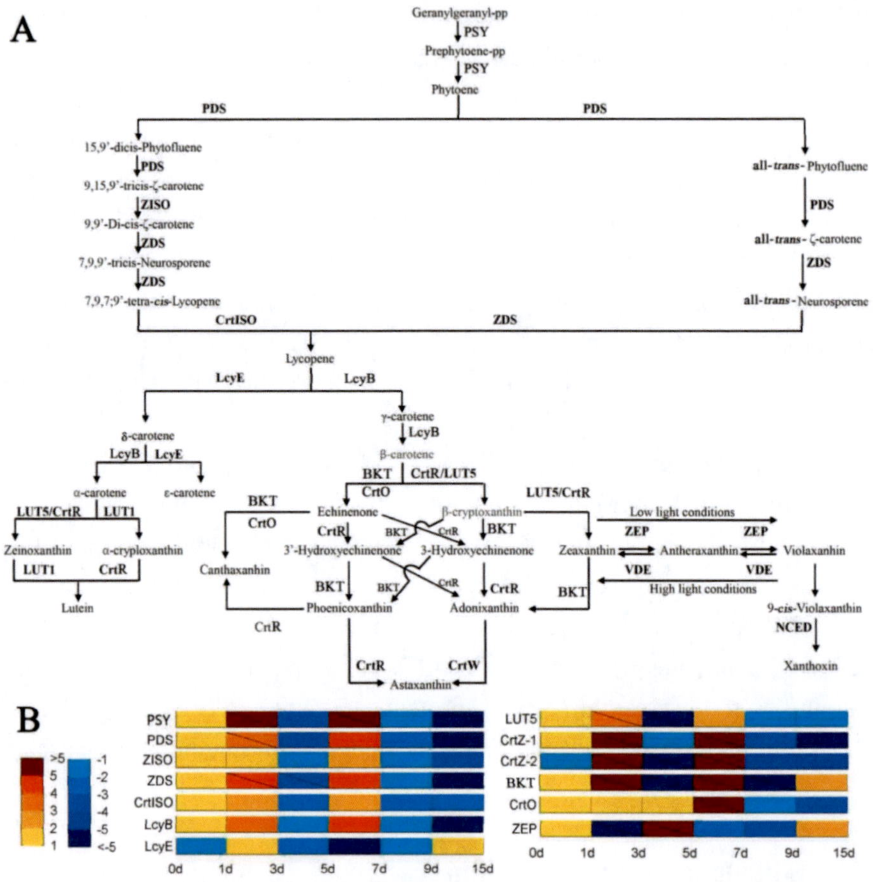

Figure 5. (A) Hypothetical carotenoid biosynthesis pathway for *Haematococcus pluvialis* generated by KEGG. Enzyme designation is according to the corresponding gene: PSY, phytoene synthase; PDS, phytoene desaturase; ZDS, ζ-carotene desaturase; ZISO; ζ-carotene isomerase; CrtISO, prolycopene isomerase; LcyE, lycopene ε-cyclase; LcyB, lycopene β-cyclase; BKT, β-carotene ketolase; CrtO, β-carotene C-4 oxygenase; LUT5, β-ring hydroxylase; LUT1, carotene ε-monooxygenase; CrtR, β-carotene 3-hydroxylase; ZEP, zeaxanthin epoxidase; VDE, violaxanthin de-epoxidase; NCED, 9-*cis*-epoxycarotenoid dioxygenase. (B) Differential expression pattern of genes involved in the carotenoid biosynthesis pathway of *Haematococcus pluvialis*. The color chart represents degree (fold) of up-(red) and down-(blue) regulation. The slash in the rectangle indicates a significant differential expression of >2 fold, $P < 0.05$ (Li et al. 2019).

Carotene ε-monooxygenase (LUT1), violaxanthin de-epoxidase (VDE), 9-*cis*-epoxycarotenoid dioxygenase (NCED) and β-carotene 3-hydroxylase (CrtR-3) were not found to be differentially expressed during cell transformation and astaxanthin accumulation. The low expression of VDE, NCED, LUT1, CrtR-3 probably was the reason for astaxanthin accumulation in *H. pluvialis*. The up-regulation of lycopene β-cyclase (LcyB) in the cell transformation was accompanied by the down-regulation of lycopene ε-cyclase (LcyE). The opposite regulation pattern of LcyB and LcyE was speculated tom be a good strategy to promote the accumulation of β-carotene, rather than δ-carotene. β-carotene ketolase (BKT) came into focus for its most extensive change, followed by CrtR-1, CrtR-2. RT-qPCR results were proved to be consistent with the transcriptomic data. BKT and CrtR were further confirmed to play an essential role in the stress-dependent initiation of astaxanthin synthesis. Based on the DEG results and KEGG pathway analysis of carotenoid synthesis overall, a hypothetical astaxanthin accumulation process in *H. pluvialis* proposed (Figure 5; Li et al. 2018).

REGULATION OF ASTAXANTHIN BIOSYNTHESIS OR CELL GROWTH

Isopentenyl pyrophosphate (IPP) is the precursor for carotenoid synthesis (Lichtenthaler 1999; Han et al. 2013). Two distinct pathways for IPP biosynthesis have been found in higher plants: the mevalonate pathway (MVA pathway) in the cytosol and the non-mevalonate 1-deoxy-D-xylulose-5-phosphate pathway in the chloroplast (DOXP pathway or MEP pathway) (Lichtenthaler et al. 1997; Han et al. 2013). In *H. pluvialis*, IPP is believed to be synthesized solely from the MEP pathway (Disch et al. 1998). Subsequently, the isopentenyl pyrophosphate isomerase (IPI) catalyzes the isomerization of IPP to dimethylallyl diphosphate (Lichtenthaler 1999). Phytoene synthase (PSY) catalyzes geranylgeranyl pyrophosphate molecules to form phytoene. Through a series of dehydrogenation reactions, two structurally similar enzymes, phytoene desaturase (PDS) and ζ-carotene desaturase (ZDS) convert the phytoene into lycopene, then to form β-carotene and astaxanthin (Cunningham and Gantt 1998; Han et al. 2013). Astaxanthin biosynthesis and cell growth of *H. pluvialis* can be regulated by other metabolic processes or signals.

Chlororespiration

Chlororespiration is a respiratory electron transport chain (ETC) by conversion of molecular oxygen into water within the thylakoid membrane of chloroplasts, and in interaction with the photosynthetic ETC (Peltier and Cournac, 2002; Cruz et al., 2011). Chlororespiration was first originally proposed by Bennoun in green algae (Bennoun 1982), and proved by redox interactions between chloroplasts and mitochondria in intact algal cells, using chlorophyll fluorescence measurements. This process is thought to involve a proton pumping NAD(P)H dehydrogenase (the NDH complex) and plastid terminal oxidase (PTOX), the former reduces the plastoquinol pool and the latter catalyzes the oxidation of the plastoquinone (PQ) pool (Rumeau et al. 2007).

The plastid terminal oxidase (PTOX) is a non-heme diiron quinol oxidase, which evolved from a common ancestral diiron carboxylate protein as well as alternative oxidase in mitochondria (McDonald and Vanlerberghe 2006). Usually, under non-stress conditions, PTOX concentrations are low possibly due to dominating linear electron transport and no access to its substrate plastoquinol (Lennon et al. 2003; Krieger-Liszkay and Feilke 2016). Under abiotic stress conditions, such as high light and high/low temperatures (Quiles 2006; Ivanov et al. 2012), salinity (Stepien and Johnson, 2009), and UV light (Laureau et al., 2013), PTOX levels elevate, because linear electron transport slow down, and the plastoquinol concentration increase, leading to PTOX associating with PQ and catalyzing the oxidation of plastoquinol (Krieger-Liszkay and Feilke 2016).

One of the important roles of PTOX is involved in carotenoid biosynthesis, due to its activity of oxidizing PQ with which to oxidize phytoene, a carotenoid intermediate. Astaxanthin biosynthesis of *H. pluvialis* derived from carotenogenesis, involving oxygenation and hydroxylation steps (Breitenbach et al. 1996; Fraser et al. 1997), in which the PDS and subsequent ζ-carotene desaturation may provide electrons to reduce the PQ pool, which in turn reduces molecular oxygen into water catalyzed by PTOX (Li et al. 2008; Gemmecker et al. 2015). Without this enzyme, the carotenoid biosynthesis slows down because of lacking oxidized PQ with which to oxidize phytoene, a colorless carotenoid, resulting in white patches of leaves (Carol and Kuntz 2001). In *Chlamydomonas reinhardtii*, PTOX possesses two isoforms, PTOX1 and PTOX2, the former is likely in charge of regenerating PQ for PDS, and the latter is the major oxidase involved in chlororespiration (Houille-Vernesetal. 2011). In *H. pluvialis*, the transcriptional expression in both genes *ptox1* and *ptox2* up-regulated transiently when algal cultures transferred from low light to high light, and the different expression patterns of these two genes shows the function of *ptox2* was coupled with carotenoid desaturation to remove excess electrons, while *ptox1* was activated only with severe or persistent stress condition (Li et al. 2008). According to the results of Western Blot (Zhang et al. 2017b), the level of PTOX protein did not change during cell transformation phase, and increased gradually during astaxanthin accumulation phase, consistent with astaxanthin accumulation of *H. pluvialis* during outdoor incubation in tubular photobioreactors.

Moreover, another important role of PTOX is photoprotection. The lack of this enzyme would cause photodamage indirectly as a result of reduced protective carotenoids (Aluru and Rodermel 2004). On the other hand, PTOX also acts as a safety valve under abiotic stress, by protecting the chloroplast ETC from over-reduction (Sun and Wen 2011), and considerably reduce formation of active oxygen species (ROS) by consumption of molecular oxygen (Li et al. 2008). However, one study showed that overexpression of PTOX promotes oxidative stress in tobacco (Heyno et al. 2009). Exposure to excess light, PTOX may have a significant role by removing excess electrons during astaxanthin accumulation in *H. pluvialis* (Zhang et al. 2017b).

In conclusion, PTOX of chlororespiration may involve in astaxanthin accumulation of *H. pluvialis* via at least two ways as following (Figure 6): (1) directly participate in the biosynthesis of astaxanthin by catalyzing the oxidation of PQ pool, which is reduced by the electron transport from carotenogenic desaturation steps. (2) act as photoprotection mechanism to promote astaxanthin accumulation indirectly, by preventing over-reduction of chloroplast ETC and reducing ROS formation from molecular oxygen.

Photorespiration

Photorespiration is considered to be a carbon cycle system (Maurino and Peterhansel 2010) and is recognized as a key ancillary component of photosynthesis (Bauwe et al. 2012). It is widely accepted that photorespiration influences bioenergetics, PSII function, and carbon metabolism to nitrogen assimilation and respiration, as well as multiple signaling pathways, particularly those that govern plant hormonal responses controlling growth, environmental and defense responses, and programmed cell death (Foyer et al. 2009). A complex network of substance metabolism and enzyme reactions occur in this process taking place in chloroplasts, peroxisomes and mitochondria. This process used to be thought as wasteful, because of potentially reducing photosynthetic output by 25% in C3 plants (Sharkey and Thomas 1988; Leegood 2007). It is a process where photosynthesis substrate Ribulose-1,5-bisphosphate (RuBP) is oxygenated rather than carboxylation by Rubisco, caused by O_2 substituting for CO_2, which results in the production of the toxic product phosphoglycolate. Photorespiration involves conversion of the phosphoglycolate to glycine, followed by the conversion of glycine to serine, and finally serine is converted to glycerate which feeds into the Calvin cycle as 3-phosphoglycerate (PGA) (Wingler et al. 2000). Therefore, photorespiration might affect the turnover of PGA.

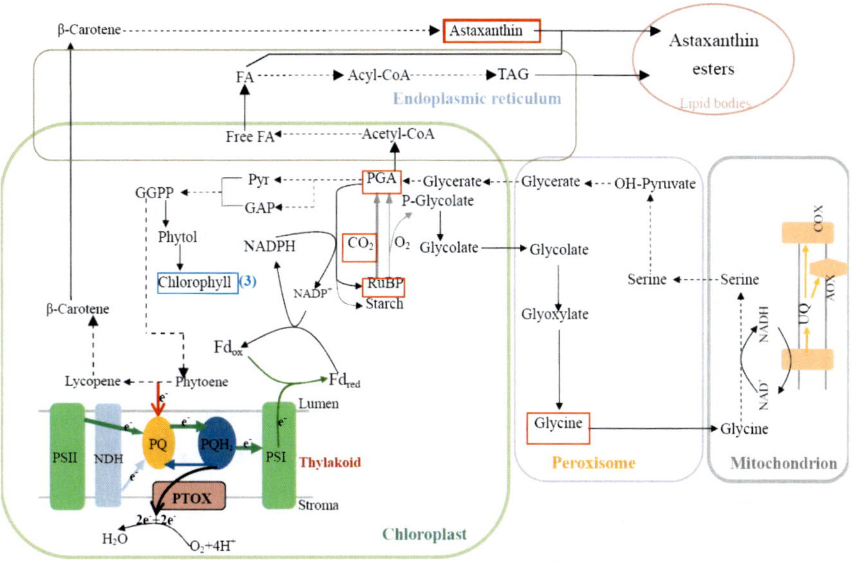

Figure 6. The relationship between astaxanthin biosynthesis and photosynthesis, chlororespiration, photorespiration, fatty acid biosynthesis. *PGA* 3-phosphoglycerate, *CEF-I* cyclic electron flow around PSI, *PSII/I* photosystem II/I, *RuBP* ribulose 1,5-biphosphate, *Rubisco* ribulose 1,5-biphosphate carboxylase/oxygenase, *GAP* glyceraldehyde-3- phosphate, *Pyr* pyruvate, *GGPP* geranylgeranyl diphosphate, Fd_{ox}/ Fd_{red} ferredoxin, *PQ* plastoquinone, *UQ* ubiquinone, *AOX* alternative oxidase, *COX* cytochrome oxidase, *NDH* NADPH dehydrogenase, *PTOX* plastid terminal oxidase, *FA* fatty acid, *TAG* triacylglycerols.

Astaxanthin derives from carotenogenesis in cytosolic lipid bodies under stress conditions (Johnson and An 1991; Johnson and Schroeder 1996). In *H. pluvialis*, the precursor of carotenoids IPP) is synthesized only by the MEP pathway in the chloroplast (Lichtenthaler et al. 1997; Disch et al. 1998; Lichtenthaler 1997). The substance 3-phosphoglyceraldehyde (GAP) and pyruvate (Pyr) are precursors to synthesize IPP in this process (Sprenger et al. 1997; Grolle et al. 2000). In addition, PGA could be converted to GAP and pyruvate (Andrews and Kane 1991). In other words, PGA is the common metabolic intermediate of the astaxanthin biosynthesis, photosynthesis and photorespiratory pathway.

In the previous study, the results showed that astaxanthin accumulation significantly decreased in *H. pluvialis* when photorespiration was inhibited by carboxymethoxylamine (CM). A detailed analysis of the process showed that the inhibition of the photorespiratory pathway would impair photosynthetic carbon assimilation (Bykova et al. 2005), with decreased actual efficiency of PSII photochemical activity (Φ_{PSII}) and attenuation of total photosynthetic rates in *H. pluvialis* (Zhang et al. 2016a). Therefore, we proposed photorespiration affect astaxanthin accumulation in *H. pluvialis* as follows (Figure 6): (1) directly enhance the accumulation of astaxanthin, by increasing the generation of PGA-conversion of the phosphoglycolate-the photorespiratory production. (2) indirectly promote astaxanthin accumulation due to increased PGA amounts by accelerating the activity of photosynthetic carbon assimilation, as photosynthetic activity was attenuation because of inhibited photorespiratory performance.

Fatty Acid

Under various environmental stress conditions, the green alga *H. pluvialis* has the capability to accumulate high amounts of astaxanthin, in cytoplasmic lipid globules (Tjahjono et al. 1994; Sarada et al. 2002), due to its ability to deposit the fatty acid- esterified pigment (Boussiba 2000). It is widely known that astaxanthin accumulation is correlated with fatty acid biosynthesis in *H. pluvialis*, while the detailed interdependence between both processes needs to be further clarified.

According to the previous study, 90% of staxanthin in *H. pluvialis* is attached with one or two fatty acids, in which (3S,3′S)-astaxanthin diester is 34%, and (3S,3′S)-astaxanthin monoester is 46%, free astaxanthin monomer is 10% (Grung et al. 1992; Miao et al. 2006). Under high light, the inhibition of fatty acid synthesis by cerulenin, resulted in the inhibition of astaxanthin accumulation in *H. pluvialis* (Schoefs et al. 2001). It is reported that intensive de novo fatty acid synthesis occurs when cells accumulate astaxanthin, and triacylglycerols (TAG) content was linearly correlated with the accumulation of astaxanthin monoesters under stress conditions (Zhekisheva et al. 2002). Furthermore, the accumulation of neutral lipids was significantly less affected with carotenogenesis inhibitors, however, de novo fatty acid synthesis as well as astaxanthin formation drastically inhibited, with lipid biosynthesis inhibitor sethoxydim, which inhibits acetyl-CoA carboxylase (Zhekisheva et al. 2005). Therefore, the astaxanthin accumulation is correlation with fatty acid biosynthesis (Chen et al. 2015).

Moreover, *H. pluvialis* has been assessed as a biodiesel feedstock, due to its potential use to produce considerable amounts of neutral lipids, among which oleic acid predominates, mainly in the form of TAG (Damiani et al. 2010). The synthesized astaxanthin molecules in *H. pluvialis* are mainly stored in subcellular structures such as lipid bodies, constituted by TAG, and the lipid bodies may protect algal cells from excess light (Lemoine and Schoefs 2010; Li et al. 2010). It is proposed that the accumulation of a certain amount of TAG is a prerequisite for the initiation of fatty acid–esterified astaxanthin accumulation in lipid globules (Zhekisheva et al. 2005). In addition, the biosynthesis of TAG requires large amounts of reducing equivalents (NADPH), which may help relax over-reduced photosynthetic ETC and then protect algal cells (Roessler 1990).

Therefore, we proposed fatty acid biosynthesis affect astaxanthin accumulation in *H. pluvialis* in two major pathways (Figure 6): (1) directly enhance the accumulation of astaxanthin, by forming fatty acid- esterified pigment, astaxanthin mono- and diesters. (2) indirectly promote astaxanthin contents by provide protection algal cells, because of accumulating fatty acid–esterified astaxanthin in lipid globules.

Auto-Signals

The possibility of auto-signals regulating the growth of *H. pluvialis* was conducted (Sun et al. 2001; Liu et al. 2004). It evidenced that some unknown substances, like auto-signals, existed in the old culture. The auto-signals could reduce the cell growth rate by decreasing the motile cell growth and inducing cell transformation from motile cells into non-motile cells. The limitation and inducement roles of the auto-signals in the old culture were cell-density-dependent. The higher the cell density was, the more the auto-signals accumulated in the old culture, which led to a heavy cell growth limitation and easy cell transformation (Sun et al. 2001).

Further studies did not support a positive connection between inorganic carbons (CO_3^{2-} or HCO_3^-) and the auto-signals. It had been suggested that the unknown were organic dissoluble substance. The DNA data and histogram of motile cells showed that the process of DNA replication in the motile cells was not inhibited, but the process of cytoplasmic division was heavily blocked by the auto-signals (Liu et al. 2004).

CULTURE MODES

Photoautotrophic Culture Mode

The principal aim of *H. pluvialis* mass culture is, of course, to produce a steady supply of high-quality astaxanthin products. Astaxanthin production is significantly dependent on two negatively correlated parameters, the total biomass production and the biomass astaxanthin content (% dry weight). Fast cell growth (increase in biomass) is usually linked to low cellular astaxanthin content. In contrast, high levels of astaxanthin accumulation are generally associated with a large decrease in the cell growth rate. Because the culture conditions for maximum growth and maximum astaxanthin content are mutually exclusive, a two-stage batch culture mode is commonly adopted for mass cultivation of *H. pluvialis*. In the first stage (also called 'green stage' because the cells are green), the cells are maintained in a nutrient-replete growth medium and exposed to low light intensity to promote biomass production. When the cells enter into the stationary growth phase, the culture is then transited into the second stage (also called 'red stage' because the cells are turning red from green) where the cells are subjected to high light intensity and nutrient deprivation to induce astaxanthin production. In addition, the production of astaxanthin and its quality are also strongly related to both the strains of *H. pluvialis* selected for cultivation (Table 1) and the culture mode used during the mass culture.

Besides the two-stage culture mode, a single-stage cultivation mode has also been tested to produce astaxanthin in flagellates of some *H. pluvialis* strains in a chemostat system (Del Río et al. 2005; 2008; García-Malea et al. 2009). Under optimal light irradiance, nutrient concentration and dilution rate, algal biomass productivities of 0.7-1.9 g L^{-1} d^{-1} were obtained, corresponding to an astaxanthin productivity of 5.6-21 mg L^{-1} d^{-1}. The technical and economic feasibilities of this single-stage culture mode for mass culture of *H. pluvialis* remain to be seen.

In Table 1, eight strains are compared in a large number of batch cultures, for their ability to accumulate astaxanthin (Liu et al. 2016). The ability of strains H3, H6, H10, and H11, to accumulate astaxanthin, appears to be significantly higher than strains H0, H2, H5, and H9. Many studies have demonstrated that *H. pluvialis* is capable of photoautotrophic, heterotrophic, and mixotrophic growth (Boussiba and Vonshak 1991; Kobayashi et al. 1992; Chen et al. 1997; Boussiba 2000; Orosa et al. 2001; Kang et al. 2005; Li et al. 2006). Each of these growth modes has culturing advantages and disadvantages.

Table 1. Astaxanthin Content in Various Strains of *H. pluvialis*, Which Were Batch Cultured on a Large Scale in Open Raceway Ponds at the Yunnan Alphy Biotech Co., Ltd (Liu et al. 2016)

Strains	Average Astaxanthin Content (% of Dry Weight)	Number of Samples	Maximum (%)	Minimum (%)	P
Total	1.99 ± 0.64	896	4.08	0.3	0.0436 < 0.05
H0	1.90 ± 0.63	174	3.59	0.3	0.014 < 0.05
H2	1.90 ± 0.61	309	3.55	0.3	0.0007 < 0.01
H3	2.24 ± 0.74	102	4.08	0.57	0.2579 > 0.05
H5	1.90 ± 0.74	30	3.31	0.57	0.0008 < 0.01
H6	2.13 ± 0.48	159	3.5	0.92	0.0024 < 0.01
H9	1.56 ± 0.65	23	2.76	0.46	0.0179 < 0.05
H10	2.16 ± 0.58	58	3.2	0.54	0.0385 < 0.05
H11	2.29 ± 0.67	18	3.99	1.03	0.0385 < 0.05

The principal advantage of using the photoautotrophic growth mode for large-scale *H. pluvialis* cultivation derives from its steady rate of production and higher astaxanthin content, required for a high-quality astaxanthin product, although specific cell growth rate is slower than that of the other modes. Photoautotrophic cultivation of *H. pluvialis* also suffers less from the contamination problems associated with the heterotrophic and mixotrophic cultivation modes. This is because there is little organic matter in the culture throughout the growth cycle, thus allowing extended periods of steady, large-scale industrial production. Currently, essentially all *H. pluvialis* cultivation companies worldwide have adapted the photoautotrophic culture mode for commercial-scale production of natural astaxanthin, regardless of the types of cultivation systems, photobioreactors (closed flat, column, or tubular photobioreactors) or open raceway ponds, or strains of *H. pluvialis* used.

Heterotrophic and Mixotrophic Culture Modes

H. pluvialis is capable of utilize organic carbon for growth in the absence of light, which provides the means of heterotrophic and mixotrophic cultivation for astaxanthin production. Under heterotrophic conditions, *H. pluvialis* grows at a relatively low growth rate (0.22 d^{-1}) and accumulates ca. 0.5% dwt of astaxanthin (Kobayashi et al. 1992). Growth and astaxanthin production can be enhanced under mixotrophic culture conditions. A final cell density of 0.9-2.65 g L^{-1} and a maximum astaxanthin content of 1-2% dwt were obtained from mixotrophic cultures of *H. pluvialis* (Chen et al. 1997; Zhang et al. 1999; Wang et al. 2004). A heterophotric-photoautotrophic culture mode was also explored where heterotrophic culture produced algal biomass, while astaxanthin production was induced during photoautotrophic culture. As a result, a very high cellular astaxanthin content of 7% by dwt, but low astaxanthin productivities of 4.4-6.5 mg L^{-1} d^{-1} were obtained (Hata et al. 2001; Kang et al. 2005).

Unfortunately, the advantages of heterotrophic cultivation of *H. pluvialis* disappear when cultivation is scaled up to achieve tons of commercial production because astaxanthin synthesis and accumulation are strongly light-induced processes for *H. pluvialis* (Steinbrenner and Linden 2000; 2003). With current knowledge and technology (e.g., the available strains), it is essentially impossible to obtain a high astaxanthin content and high-quality astaxanthin products using heterotrophic metabolism, without subjecting the cells to a follow-up growth period under photosynthetic, photoautotrophic, and/or mixotrophic, cultivation. A further complication is that during such a secondary phototrophic cultivation period for astaxanthin accumulation, especially in large-scale cultivation, it is nearly impossible to maintain an axenic culture of *H. pluvialis*. Unwanted microorganisms (including fungi, bacteria, and other species of microalgae) invade the system from various sources and quickly multiply using the residual organic materials remaining after the heterotrophic growth stage, inevitably reducing the quality of the final products. Contamination with algal-grazing zooplankton can even destroy the entire *H. pluvialis* culture.

Large-scale mixotrophic culture of *H. pluvialis* faces similar shortcomings and problems as those just described for the heterotrophic culture approach. The advantage for mixotrophic culturing, which is to obtain high biomass production and astaxanthin accumulation in small-scale cultures, vanishes on scale-up due to the inevitable culture-contamination issue. For heterotrophic or mixotrophic approaches to be useful for large-scale cultivation of *H. pluvialis*, a break-through in contamination control will be required.

Heterotrophic-Phototrophic Culture Mode

Recently, a new paradigm that integrated heterotrophic cultivation, acclimation of heterotrophically grown cells to specific light/nutrient regimes, followed by induction of astaxanthin accumulation under photoautotrophic conditions was developed (Zhang et al. 2016b). First, the environmental conditions such as pH, carbon source, nitrogen regime, and light intensity, were optimized to induce astaxanthin accumulation in the dark-grown cells. To minimize the susceptibility of dark-grown *H. pluvialis* cells to light stress, the algal cells were acclimated, prior to light induction of astaxanthin biosynthesis, under moderate illumination in the presence of nitrogen. Introduction of this strategy significantly reduced the cell mortality rate under high-light and resulted in increased astaxanthin productivity. The productivity of astaxanthin was further improved significantly by implementation of such a strategy in a bubbling column photobioreactor (Zhang et al. 2016b).

The new culture strategy is developed to mitigate the death of heterotrophy-grown cells in the process of high-light induction of astaxanthin accumulation, which significantly increased the astaxanthin productivity as a consequence. Along with a combination of heterotrophy and autotrophy cultivation modes for biomass and astaxanthin production, respectively, this strategy is promising for commercial-scale astaxanthin production in the future (Zhang et al. 2016b).

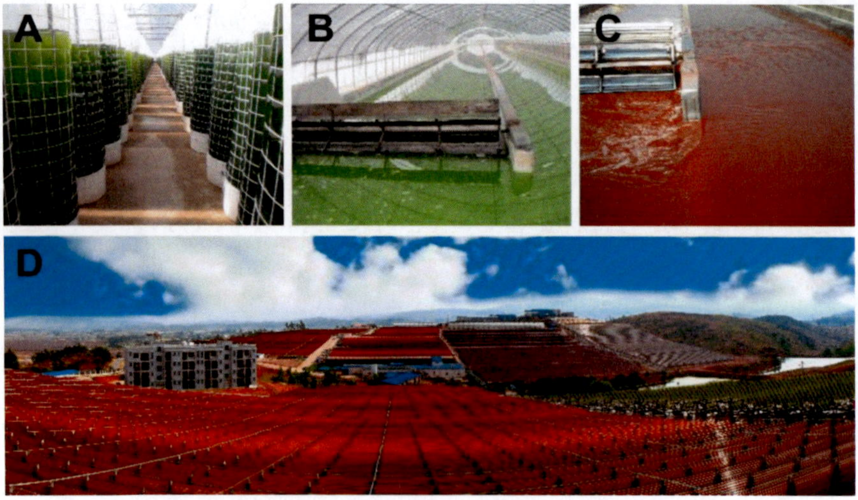

Figure 7. Photobioreactors used for industrial-scale production of *Haematococcus pluvialis*. (a) closed column photobioreactors inside a greenhouse; (b) open raceway pond inside a greenhouse; (c) open raceway pond outdoors; and (d) closed tubular photobioreactors outdoors.

PHOTOBIOREACTORS

H. pluvialis were mass-scale cultivated using a two-stage culturing technique (Han et al. 2013; Liu et al. 2016). The algae were first cultured in photobioreactors for fast cell growth and high biomass. When the biomass reached its maximum, cell cultures were transferred into stress environmental conditions to induce cell transformation from motile cells to non-motile cells. Then, the non-motile cells started to accumulate astaxanthin in the closed tubular photobioreactors and/or open runway ponds.

Many types of photobioreactors have been developed in the past decades. The most widely used closed photobioreactors include flat-, column-, and tubular designs (Liu et al. 2016). Those used for outdoor mass-cultivation rather than indoor basic scientific studies, have the advantage of using free solar energy to drive the growth of photoautotrophic cultures. Up to now, no single photobioreactor, no matter its type, possesses all the characteristics desired for industrial cultivation of *H. pluvialis*. Each type of photobioreactors has its own advantages and disadvantages. For example, precise-control photobioreactors, in which most of the culture parameters can be monitored and controlled, is that they can maintain a fast cell growth and high cell density. However, their shortcomings are that they are expensive and usually of small size. Thus, such a precise-control photobioreactor could only be used for laboratory studies or for indoor cultivation to obtain a pure, dense inoculum for initiating cultivation in larger vessels. Selecting an appropriate mix of photobioreactors that have various strengths and can compensate for each other's weaknesses is an important issue in large-scale cultivation, as this approach can result in a reliable and smooth scale-up of the starter culture to industrial scale. Comparative studies based on actual situations should be performed to get information that would allow a balanced decision about such infrastructure. Closed column photobioreactors and tubular photobioreactors, as well as open raceway ponds have been selected for use in our two-stage cultivation of *H. pluvialis* for astaxanthin production in Yunnan Province of China (Figure 7; Liu et al. 2016).

Control of Biological Contamination

Sustained production of natural astaxanthin is dependent not only on the technologies promoting cell growth and accelerating astaxanthin accumulation but also on the effectiveness of protecting the culture from biological contamination. Usually, However, during the scale-up of cultures, especially for outdoor mass cultivation of *H. pluvialis*, biological contaminants inevitably infect the cultures through various routes, whether in open raceway ponds or in closed photobioreactors. Most of the contaminating organisms generally become much more active and multiply rapidly at a moderately high temperature; therefore, biological contamination is a particularly serious problem during the hot and rainy seasons. Biological contamination reduces the cell growth rate and decreases the astaxanthin content in the biomass (Liu et al. 2016).

Mass culture of *H. pluvialis* can be contaminated by many species of microorganism from bacteria and fungi to species of fast-growing microalgae, as well as grazers (rotifers, amoebae, protozoa, etc.), resulting in reduced biomass yield and quality, and sometimes loss of culture all together. These contaminants can enter and infect cultures through nutrient and water addition, gas (air and CO_2) bubbling, incompletely sterilized culture devices, insufficient care during culture manipulation, and even a contaminated inoculum. For example, a parasitic blastoclad fungus identified as *Paraphysoderma sedebokerensis* is the most devastating disease responsible for reduced astaxanthin productivity and frequent culture collapses (Hoffman et al. 2008; Gutman et al. 2009). Hoffman et al. (2008) made detailed observations on the infection of *H. pluvialis* culture by the parasite *P. sedebokerensis* (Hoffman et al. 2008). During the infection process, healthy green culture turns dark brown, accompanied by the formation of large clumps consisting of living cells, cell debris, and particulate organic matters. A more vivid red color of culture can be first observed if infection occurred at the red stage, followed by gradual bleaching of algal cells (Hoffman et al. 2008).

At present, methods of physical prevention (thermal sterilization, micropore filtration, UV radiation, etc.) are the best options. Chemical control agents (some reagents and synthetic chemical pesticides) are only feasible in small-scale cultures of *H. pluvialis*; none of these is sufficiently safe, selective, and effective to deal with biological contamination in large-scale cultures.

Comprehensive methods to avoid biological contamination of cultures during the process of biomass expansion remain the most crucial technology (perhaps exceeding the importance of all other culture aspects) in commercial production of *H. pluvialis* for astaxanthin. These integrated technical methods include thorough sterilization or disinfection of culture devices; strict aseptic technique; well-trained process control and management personnel; minimization of contamination opportunities, particularly during the early culture stage; effective amplification of the axenic monoculture volume by using closed photobioreactors; and skilled control of parameters that enhance cell density and keep the culture in a fast, logarithmic, cell growth phase and provide high-quality algal cells for the inoculum. In addition, timely detection and efficient elimination of any biological contaminants that do get into the cultures are primary tasks for daily management and process control. Early detection and treatment reduce the probability of a rapid and extensive proliferation of the biological contaminants, which otherwise might lead to more wide-spread contamination of the surrounding environment and initiate a vicious cycle of contaminations. Drugs that inhibit biological contaminants without damaging the nontarget microalgae are the preferred treatment choices when physical control measures fail. Biopesticides are a good alternative, owing to their effectiveness and relatively safe properties (Huang et al. 2014a,b). Finding and developing some efficient and highly selective natural pesticides that can take the place of broad-spectrum pesticides that also have low toxicity to *H. pluvialis* cells, and degrade rapidly without affecting the quality of products, is another important subject for ongoing studies. Successful selection of such substances is a major challenge for phycologists but has a great potential for industrial application. Then, the development of various, effective, closed photobioreactors, and using them in conjunction with appropriate natural pesticides, should be an effective approach for controlling contaminants in mass cultivation of *H. pluvialis*.

Perspectives

Astaxanthin accumulation in *H. pluvialis* interacts with multiple metabolic pathways. However, the molecular mechanisms mediating the crosstalk between astaxanthin accumulation and related metabolic pathways need to further illuminate. Commercial farming of *H. pluvialis*, an excellent source of natural astaxanthin, shows considerable promise with commercial-scale production already ongoing in several countries. Mass cultivation of *H. pluvialis* is already physically and economically feasible and profitable, and this industry is bound to expand in the near future.

References

Aluru MR, Rodermel SR. 2004. Control of chloroplast redox by the IMMUTANS terminal oxidase. *Physiol. Plant.* 120: 4-11.

Andrews TJ, Kane HJ. 1991. Pyruvate is a by-product of catalysis by ribulosebisphosphate carboxylase/oxygenase. *J. Biolo. Chem.* 266: 9447-9452.

Bauwe H, Hagemann M, Kern R, Timm S. 2012. Photorespiration has a dual origin and manifold links to central metabolism. *Curr. Opin. plant biolo.* 15: 269-275.

Benemann, JR. 1992. Microalgae aquaculture feeds. *J. Appl. Phycol.* 4: 233-245.

Bennoun P. 1982. Evidence for a respiratory chain in the chloroplast. *Proc. Natl Acad. Sci. USA* 79: 4352-4356.

Bernhard K. 1990. Synthetic Astaxanthin. The Route of a Carotenoid from Research to Commercialisation. In: Krinsky NI et al. Eds, *Carotenoids: Chemistry and Biology.* Springer, New York, US, pp 337-363.

Boussiba S. 2000. Carotenogenesis in the green alga *Haematococcus pluvialis*: Cellular physiology and stress response. *Physiol. Plant.* 108: 111-117.

Boussiba S, Bing W, Yuan JP, Zarka A, Chen F. 1999. Changes in pigments profile in the green alga *Haeamtococcus pluvialis* exposed to environmental stresses. *Biotechnol. Lett.* 21: 601-604.

Boussiba S, Vonshak A. 1991. Astaxanthin accumulation in the green alga *Haematococcus pluvialis*. *Plant Cell Physiol.* 32: 1077-1082.

Breitenbach J, Misawa N, Kajiwara S, Sandmann G. 1996. Expression in *Escherichia coli* and properties of the carotene ketolase from *Haematococcus pluvialis*. *FEMS Microbiol. Lett.* 140: 241-246.

Bykova NV, Keerberg O, Pärnik T, Bauwe H, Gardeström P. 2005. Interaction between photorespiration and respiration in transgenic potato plants with antisense reduction in glycine decarboxylase. *Planta* 222: 130-140.

Carol P, Kuntz M. 2001. A plastid terminal oxidase comes to light: implications for carotenoid biosynthesis and chlororespiration. *Trends Plant Sci.* 6: 31-36.

Chen G. 2007. *Lipid and fatty acid composition and their biosyntheses in relation to carotenoid accumulation in the microalgae Nitzschia laevis (Bacillariophyceae) and Haematococcus pluvialis (Chlorophyceae).* PhD dissertation, The University of Hong Kong, Hong Kong, pp 150.

Chen GQ, Wang BB, Han DX, Sommerfeld M, Lu YH, Chen F, Hu Q. 2015. Molecular mechanisms of the coordination between astaxanthin and fatty acid biosynthesis in *Haematococcus pluvialis* (Chlorophyceae). *Plant J.* 81: 95-107.

Chen H, Chen F, Dong, XD. 1997. Mixotrophic and heterotrophic growth of *Haematococcus lacustris* and rheological behaviour of the cell suspensions. *Bioresour. Technol.* 1: 19-24.

Cruz S, Goss R, Wilhelm C, Leegood R, Horton P, Jakob T, Notes A. 2011. Impact of chlororespiration on non-photochemical quenching of chlorophyll fluorescence and on the regulation of the diadinoxanthin cycle in the diatom *Thalassiosira pseudonana*. *J. Exp. Bot.* 62: 509-519.

Cunningham FX, Gantt E. 1998. Genes and enzymes of carotenoid biosynthesis in plants. *Annu. Rev. Plant Physiol. Plant Mol. Biol.* 49: 557-583.

Damiani MC, Popovich CA, Constenla D, Leonardi PI. 2010. Lipid analysis in *Haematococcus pluvialis* to assess its potential use as a biodiesel feedstock. *Bioresour. Technol.* 101: 3801-3807.

Del Río E, Acién FG, García-Malea MC, Rivas J, Moli-na-Grima E, Guerrero MG. 2008. Efficiency assessment of the one-step production of astaxanthin by the microalga *Haematococcus pluvialis*. *Biotechnol. Bioeng.* 100: 397-402.

Del Río E, Acién FG, García-Malea MC, Rivas J, Molina-Grima E, Guerrero MG. 2005. Efficient one-step production of astaxanthin by the microalga *Haematococcus pluvialis* in continuous culture. *Biotechnol. Bioeng.* 91: 808-815.

Disch A, Schwender J, Müller C, Lichtenthaler HK, Rohmer M. 1998. Distribution of the mevalonate and glyceraldehyde phosphate/pyruvate pathways for isoprenoid biosynthesis in unicellular algae and the cyanobacterium *Synechocystis* PCC 6714. *Biochem. J.* 333: 381-388.

Doering W, Leventis C, Roth W. 1995. Thermal inter -conversions among 15-cis-, 13-cis-, and all-trans-β-carotene: kinetics, arrhenius parameters, thermo -chemistry, and potential relevance to anti-carcinogenicity of all-trans-β-carotene. *J. Am. Chem. Soc.* 117: 2747-2757.

Elliot AM. 1934. Morphology and life history of *Haematococcus pluvialis*. *Arch. Protistenk.* 82: 250-272.

Foyer CH, Bloom AJ, Queval G, Noctor G. 2009. Photorespiratory Metabolism: Genes, Mutants, Energetics, and Redox Signaling. *Annu. Rev. Plant Biol.* 60: 455-484.

Fraser PD, Miura Y, Misawa N. 1997. *In vitro* characterization of astaxanthin biosynthetic enzymes. *J. Biol. Chem.* 272: 6128-6135.

Gao G, Wei CC, Jeevarajan AS, Kispert LD. 1996. Geometrical Isomerization of Carotenoids Mediated by Cation Radical/Dication Formation. *J. Phys. Chem.* 100: 5362-5366.

García-Malea MC, Acién FG, Del Río E, Fernández JM, Cerón MC, Guerrero MG, Molina-Grima E. 2009. Production of astaxanthin by *Haematococcus pluvialis* taking the one-step system outdoors. *Biotechnol. Bioeng.* 102: 651-657.

Gemmecker S, Schaub P, Koschmieder J, Brausemann A, Drepper F, Rodriguez-Franco M, Ghisla S, Warscheid B, Einsle O, Beyer P. 2015. Phytoene Desaturase from *Oryza sativa*: Oligomeric Assembly, Membrane Association and Preliminary 3d-Analysis. *PloS ONE* 10: e0131717.

Giannelli L, Yamada H, Katsuda T, Yamaji H. 2015. Effects of temperature on the astaxanthin productivity and light harvesting characteristics of the green alga *Haematococcus pluvialis*. *J. Biosci. Bioeng.* 119: 345-350.

Goswami G, Chaudhuri S, Dutta D. 2010. The present perspective of astaxanthin with reference to biosynthesis and pharmacological importance. *World J. Microbiol. Biotechnol.* 26: 1925-1939.

Grolle S, Bringer-Meyer S, Sahm H. 2000. Isolation of the dxr gene of *Zymomonas mobilis* and characterization of the 1-deoxy-D-xylulose 5-phosphate reductoisomerase. *FEMS Microbiol. Lett.* 191: 131-137.

Grung M, Dsouza FML, Borowitzka M, Liaaenjensen S. 1992. Algal carotenoids 51. secondary carotenoids 2. *Haematococcus pluvialis* aplanospores as a source of (3s, 3's)-astaxanthin esters. *J. Appl. Phycol.* 4: 165-171.

Guang Z. 2008. Plant Chlorophyll Degradation. *Plant Physiol. Communications* 44: 7-14.

Guerin M, Huntley ME, Olaizola M. 2003. *Haematococcus* astaxanthin: Applications for human health and nutrition. *Trends Biotechnol.* 21: 210-216.

Gutman J, Zarka A, Boussiba S. 2009. The host-range of *Paraphysoderma sedebokerensis*, a chytrid that infects *Haematococcus pluvialis*. *Eur. J. Phycol.* 44: 509-514.

Han DX, Li YT, Hu Q. 2013. Astaxanthin in microalgae: pathways, functions and biotechnological implications. *Algae* 28: 131-147.

Harker M, Tsavalos A, Young A. 1996. Autotrophic growth and carotenoid production of *Haematococcus pluvialis*, in a 30 liter air-lift photobioreactor. *J. Ferment. Bioeng.* 82: 113-118.

Hata N, Ogbonna JC, Hasegawa Y, Taroda H, Tanaka H. 2001. Production of astaxanthin by *Haematococcus pluvialis* in a sequential heterotrophic-photoautotrophic culture. *J. Appl. Phycol.* 13: 395-402.

Heyno E, Gross CM, Laureau C, Culcasi M, Pietri S, Krieger-Liszkay A. 2009. Plastid alternative oxidase (PTOX) promotes oxidative stress when overexpressed in tobacco. *J. Biol. Chem.* 284: 31174-31180.

Hoffman Y, Aflalo C, Zarka A, Gutman J, James TY, Boussiba S. 2008. Isolation and characterization of a novel chytrid species (phylum Blastocladiomycota), parasitic on the green alga *Haermatococcus. Mycol. Res.* 112: 70-81.

Houille-Vernes L, Rappaport F, Wollman F, Alric J, Johnson X. 2011. Plastid terminal oxidase 2 (PTOX2) is the major oxidase involved in chlororespiration in *Chlamydomonas*. *Proc. Natl. Acad. Sci. USA* 108: 20820-20825.

Huang Y, Liu JG, Li L, Tong P, Zhang LT. 2014b. Efficacy of binary combinations of botanical pesticides for rotifer elimination in microalgal cultivation. *Bioresour. Technol.* 154: 67-73.

Huang Y, Li L, Liu JG, Lin W. 2014a. Botanical pesticides as potential rotifer control agents in microalgal mass culture. *Algal Res.* 4: 62-69.

Ivanov AG, Rosso D, Savitch LV, Stachula P, Rosembert M, Oquist G, Hurry V, Hüner NPA. 2012. Implications of alternative electron sinks in increased resistance of PSII and PSI photochemistry to high light stress in cold-acclimated *Arabidopsis thaliana*. *Photosyn. Res.* 113: 191-206.

Johnson EA, An GH. 1991. Astaxanthin from microbial sources. *Crit. Rev. Biotechnol.* 11: 297-326.

Johnson EA, Schroeder WA. 1996. Biotechnology of astaxanthin production in Phaffia rhodozyma. In: Takeda GR, Teranishi R, Williams PJ Eds, *Biotechnology for Improved Foods and Flavors*. American Chemical Society, pp 39-50.

Kang CD, Lee JS, Park TH, Sim SJ. 2005. Comparison of heterotrophic and photoautotrophic induction on astaxanthin production by *Haematococcus pluvialis*. *Appl. Microbiol. Biotechnol.* 68: 237-241.

Kobayashi M, Sakamoto Y. 1999. Singlet oxygen quenching ability of astaxanthin esters from the green alga *Haematococcus pluvialis*. *Biotechnol. Lett.* 21: 265-269.

Kobayashi M. 2000. *In vivo* antioxidant role of astaxanthin under oxidative stress in the green alga *Haematococcus pluvialis*. *Appl. Microbiol. Biotechnol.* 54: 550-555.

Kobayashi M. 2003. Astaxanthin biosynthesis enhanced by reactive oxygen species in the green alga *Haematococcus pluvialis*. *Biotechnol. Bioproc. E.* 8: 322-330.

Kobayashi M, Kakizono T, Nishio N, Nagai S. 1992. Effects of light intensity, light quality, and illumination cycle on astaxanthin formation in a green alga, *Haematococcus pluvialis*. *J. Ferment. Bioeng.* 74: 61-63.

Krieger-l-Liszkay A, Feilke K. 2016. The Dual Role of the Plastid Terminal Oxidase PTOX: Between a Protective and a Pro-oxidant Function. *Front. Plant Sci.* 6(9): 1147.

Laureau C, De Paepe R, Latouche G, Moreno-Chacón M, Finazzi G, Kuntz M, Cornic G, Streb P. 2013. Plastid terminal oxidase (PTOX) has the potential to act as a safety valve for excess excitation energy in the alpine plant species *Ranunculus glacialis* L. *Plant Cell Environ.* 36: 1296-1310.

Leegood RC. 2007. A welcome diversion from photorespiration. *Nature Biotechnol.* 25: 539-540.

Lemoine Y, Schoefs B. 2010. Secondary ketocarotenoid astaxanthin biosynthesis in algae: a multifunctional response to stress. *Photosynth. Res.* 106: 155-177.

Lennon AM, Prommeenate P, Nixon PJ. 2003. Location, expression and orientation of the putative chlororespiratory enzymes, ndh andimmutans, in higher-plant plastids. *Planta* 218: 254-260.

Leya T, Rahn A, Lütz C, Remias D. 2009. Response of arctic snow and permafrost algae to high light and nitrogen stress by changes in pigment composition and applied aspects for biotechnology. *FEMS Microbiol. Ecol.* 67: 432-443.

Li QQ, Zhang LT, Liu JG. 2019. Comparative transcriptome analysis at seven time points during *Haematococcus pluvialis* motile cell growth and astaxanthin accumulation. *Aquaculture* 503: 304-311.

Li Y, Sommerfeld M, Chen F, Hu Q. 2010. Effect of photon flux densities on regulation of carotenogenesis and cell viability of Haematococcus pluvialis (Chlorophyceae*). J. Appl. Phycol.* 22: 253-263.

Li YT, Sommerfeld M, Chen F, Hu Q. 2008. Consumption of oxygen by astaxanthin biosynthesis: A protective mechanism against oxidative stress in *Haematococcus pluvialis* (Chlorophyceae). *J. Plant Physiol.* 165:1783-1797.

Li YY, Liu JG, Lin W, Cui XJ, Xue YB. 2006. Effects of light intensity on cell transformation, astaxanthin accumulation in three strains of *Haematococcus pluvialis* and their difference. *Mar. Sci*. 30: 36-41.

Lichtenthaler HK, Rohmer M, Schwender J. 1997. Two independent biochemical pathways for isopentenyl diphosphate and isoprenoid biosynthesis in higher plants. *Physiol. Plant.* 101: 643-652.

Lichtenthaler, HK. 1999. The 1-deoxy-D-xylulose-5-phosphate pathway of isoprenoid biosynthesis in plants. *Annu. Rev. Plant Physiol. Plant Mol. Biol.* 50: 47-65.

Liu X, Osawa T. 2007. Cis astaxanthin and especially 9-cis astaxanthin exhibits a higher antioxidant activity *in vitro* compared to the all-trans isomer. *Biochem. Bioph. Res. Co.* 357: 187.

Liu JG, Sun YN, Yin MY, Liu W, Zhang Z. 2004. Inorganic carbon and the cell growth regulator in *Haematococcus pluvialis*. Oceanol. Limnol. Sin. 35: 87-94 (in Chinese with English abstract, English version in *Proc. China Assoc. Sci. Technol.* 2: 454-461).

Liu JG, van der Meer JP, Zhang LT, Zhang Y. 2016. Cultivation of *Haematococcus pluvialis* for astaxanthin production. In: Slocombe SP, Benemann JR, Eds, *Micro-Algal Production for Biomass and High-Value Products;* Taylor & Francis: New York, USA, pp 267-293.

Liu JG, Zhang XL, Sun YH, Lin W. 2010. Antioxidative capacity and enzyme activity in *Haematococcus pluvialis* cells exposed to superoxide free radicals. *Chin. J. Oceanol. Limnol.* 28: 1-9.

Maurino VG, Peterhansel C. 2010. Photorespiration: current status and approaches for metabolic engineering. *Curr. Opin. Plant Biol.* 13: 248-255.

McDonald AE, Vanlerberghe GC. 2006. Origins, evolutionary history, and taxonomic distribution of alternative oxidase and plastoquinol terminal oxidase. *Comp. Biochem. Physiol. Part D Genomics Proteomics* 1: 357-364.

Miao FP, Lu DY, Li YG, Zeng MT. 2006. Characterization of astaxanthin esters in *Haematococcus pluvialis* by liquid chromatography-atmospheric pressure chemical ionization mass spectrometry. *Anal. Biochem.* 352: 176-181.

Mittler, R. 2002. Oxidative stress, antioxidants and stress tolerance. *Trends Plant Sci.* 7: 405-410.

Niyogi KK. 2000. Safety valves for photosynthesis. *Curr. Opin. Plant Biol.* 3: 455-460.

Orosa M, Franqueira D, Cid A, Abalde, J. 2001. Carotenoid accumulation in *Haematococcus pluvialis* in mixotrophic growth. *Biotechnol. Lett.* 23: 373-378.

Orosa M, Torres E, Fidalgo P, Abalde J. 2000. Production and analysis of secondary carotenoids in green algae. *J. Appl. Phycol.* 12: 553-556.

Peltier G, Cournac L. 2002. *Chlororespiration. Annu. Rev. Plant Biol.* 53: 523-550.

Quiles MJ. 2006. Stimulation of chlororespiration by heat and high light intensity in oat plants. *Plant Cell Environ.* 29:1463-1470.

Remias, D, Lütz-Meindl, U, Lütz, C. 2005. Photosynthesis, pigments and ultrastructure of the alpine snow alga *Chlamydomonas nivalis*. *Eur. J. Phycol.* 40: 259-268.

Roessler PG. 1990. Environmental control of glycerolipid metabolism in microalgae commercial implications and future research directions. *J. Phycol.* 26: 393-399.

Rumeau D, Peltier G, Cournac L. 2007. Chlororespiration and cyclic electron flow around PSI during photosynthesis and plant stress response. *Plant Cell Environ.* 30: 1041-1051.

Sarada R, Bhattacharya S, Ravishankar G. 2002. Optimization of culture conditions for growth of the green alga *Haematococcus pluvialis*. *World J. Microbial. Biotech.* 18: 517-521.

Schoefs B, Rmiki NE, Rachadi J, Lemoine Y. 2001. Astaxanthin accumulation in Haematococcus requires a cytochrome P450 hydroxylase and an active synthesis of fatty acids. *FEbs Lett.* 500: 125-128.

Sharkey TD. 1988. Estimating the rate of photorespiration in leaves. *Physiolo. Plant.* 73: 147-152.

Sommer TR, Potts WT, Morrissy NM. 1991. Utilization of microalgal astaxanthin by rainbow trout (*Oncorhyncus mykiss*). *Aquaculture* 94: 79-88.

Sprenger GA, Schorken U, Wiegert T, Grolle S, de Graaf AA, Taylor SV, Begley TP, Bringer-Meyer S, Sahm H. 1997. Identification of a thiamin-dependent synthase in *Escherichia coli* required for the formation of the 1-deoxy-D-xylulose 5-phosphate precursor to isoprenoids, thiamin, and pyridoxol. *Proc. Natl. Acad. Sci. USA* 94: 12857-12862.

Steinbrenner J, Linden H. 2003. Light induction of carotenoid biosynthesis genes in the green alga *Haematococcus pluvialis*: Regulation by photosynthetic redox control. *Plant Mol. Biol.* 52: 343-356.

Steinbrenner J, Linden H. 2000. Regulation of two carotenoid biosynthesis genes coding for phytoene synthase and carotenoid hydroxylase during stress-induced astaxanthin biosynthesis in the green alga *Haematococcus pluvialis*. *Plant Physiol.* 125: 810-817.

Stepien P, Johnson GN. 2009. Contrasting responses of photosynthesis to salt stress in the glycophyte Arabidopsis and the halophyte thellungiella: Role of the plastid terminal oxidase as an alternative electron sink. *Plant Physiol.* 149: 1154-1165.

Sun X, Wen T. 2011. Physiological roles of plastid terminal oxidase in plant stress responses. *J. Biosci.* 36: 951-956.

Sun, YN, Yin MY, Liu JG. 2001. Auto-signals in Haematococcus pluvialis. *Trans. Oceanol. Limnol.* 89: 22-28 (in Chinese with English abstract).

Tjahjono, A, Hayama, Y, Kakizono, T, Terada, Y, Nishio, N, Nagai, S. 1994. Hyper-accumulation of astaxanthin in a greenalga *Haematococcus pluvialis* at elevated temperature. *Biotechnol. Lett.* 16: 133-138.

Tsuchiya T, Ohta H, Okawa K, Iwamatsu A, Shimada H, Masuda T, Takamiya K. 1999. Cloning of chlorophyllase, the key enzyme in chlorophyll degradation: Finding of a lipase motif and the induction by methyl jasmonate. *Proc. Natl. Acad. Sci. USA* 96: 15362-15367.

Wang JF, Han DX, Sommerfeld MR, Lu CM, Hu Q. 2013. Effect of initial biomass density on growth and astaxanthin production of *Haematococcus pluvialis* in an outdoor photobioreactor. *J. Appl. Phycol.* 25: 253-260.

Wang SB, Chen F, Sommerfeld M, Hu Q. 2004. Proteomic analysis of molecular response to oxidative stress by the green alga *Haematococcus pluvialis* (Chlorophyceae). *Planta* 220: 17-29.

Wingler A, Lea PJ, Quick WP, Leegood RC. 2000. Photorespiration: metabolic pathways and their role in stress protection. *Philos. T. R. Soc. B- Biological Sciences* 355: 1517-1529.

Yang S, Zhang T, Jie XU. 2015. Chiral Separation and Analysis of Astaxanthin Stereoisomers in Biological Organisms by High-Performance Liquid Chromatography. *Food Sci.* 8: 139-144 (in Chinese with English abstract)

Zhang CH, Liu JG, Zhang LT. 2017a. Cell cycles and proliferation patterns in Haematococcus pluvialis. *Chin. J. Oceanol. Limnol.* 35: 1205-1211.

Zhang CH, Zhang LT, Liu JG. 2016a. The role of photorespiration during astaxanthin accumulation in *Haematococcus pluvialis* (Chlorophyceae). *Plant Physiol. Biochem.* 107: 75-81.

Zhang LT, Su F, Zhang CH, Gong F, Liu J. 2017b. Changes of photosynthetic behaviors and photoprotection during cell transformation and astaxanthin accumulation in *Haematococcus pluvialis* grown outdoors in tubular photobioreactors. *Int. J. Molec. Sci.* 18: 33.

Zhang Z, Wang BB, Hu Q, Sommerfeld M, Li YG, Han DX. 2016b. A new paradigm for producing astaxanthin from the unicellular green alga *Haematococcus pluvialis*. *Biotechnol. Bioeng.* 113: 2088-2099.

Zhang LT, Zhang ZS, Gao HY, Xue ZC, Yang C, Meng XL, Meng QW. 2011. Mitochondrial alternative oxdiase pathway protects plants against photoinhibition by alleviating inhibition of the repair of photodamaged PSII through preventing formation of reactive oxygen species in *Rumex* K-1 leaves. *Physiol. Plant.* 143: 396-407.

Zhang XW, Gong XD, Chen F. 1999. Kinetic models for astaxanthin production by high cell density mixotrophic culture of the microalga *Haematococcus pluvialis*. *J. Ind. Microbiol. Biotechnol.* 23: 691-696.

Zhekisheva M, Boussiba S, Khozin-Goldberg I, Zarka A, Cohen Z. 2002. Accumulation of oleic acid in *Haematococcus pluvialis* (Chlorophyceae) under nitrogen starvation or high light is correlated with that of astaxanthin eaters. *J. Phycol.* 38: 325-331.

Zhekisheva M, Zarka A, Khozin-Goldberg I, Cohen Z, Boussiba S. 2005. Inhibition of astaxanthin synthesis under high irradiance does not abolish triacylglycerol accumulation in the green alga *Haematococcus pluvialis* (Chlorophyceae). *J. Phycol.* 41: 819-826.

In: An Essential Guide to Astaxanthin ISBN: 978-1-53615-571-6
Editor: Paul A. Melborne

Chapter 3

METHODS FOR Z-ISOMERIZATION OF ASTAXANTHIN AND EFFECTS OF THE CONVERSION ON THE PHYSICOCHEMICAL PROPERTIES AND FUNCTIONALITIES

Masaki Honda*

Faculty of Science and Technology, Meijo University, Nagoya, Japan

ABSTRACT

Astaxanthin, a pigment that belongs to the family of xanthophylls, has a large number of geometric isomers due to the presence of numerous conjugated double bonds in the molecule. A number of studies have addressed that *Z*-isomers of astaxanthin would have a higher bioavailability and show a higher antioxidant capacity than the all-*E*-isomer. Hence, it is important to understand efficient *Z*-isomerization method for (all-*E*)-astaxanthin. Furthermore, very recently, several experiments have shown that the *Z*-isomerization of carotenoids including astaxanthin induced the changes in the physicochemical properties such

* Corresponding Author's E-mail: honda@meijo-u.ac.jp.

as solubility and crystallinity. It is considered that the changes in physicochemical properties of carotenoids by the *Z*-isomerization would be closely involved in the changes of the functionalities, and an accurate understanding of the relationship could contribute to fully exerting the health benefits of astaxanthin. The objective of this contribution is to review methods for *Z*-isomerization of astaxanthin and subsequent changes in the physicochemical properties and functionalities.

Keywords: carotenoid, astaxanthin, *E*/*Z*-isomerization, antioxidant capacity, bioavailability, solubility, crystallinity

INTRODUCTION

Astaxanthin is a dark-red xanthophyll carotenoid containing 13 conjugated double bonds, and is found abundantly in various microorganisms and *marine* animals (Ambati et al., 2014). In recent years, astaxanthin has attracted increasing attention because it can significantly reduce the risk of cancer and cardiovascular disease (Visioli and Artaria, 2017; Zhang and Wang, 2015), and shows an especially storong antioxidant capacity among carotenoids (Ouchi et al., 2010). Astaxanthin has a large number of geometric isomers as a result of *E*/*Z* isomerization at arbitrary sites among the multiple conjugated double bonds (Figure 1). In general, astaxanthin occur predominantly in the all-*E*-isomer in nature, whereas the *Z*-isomers are present in human body in considerable quantity, e.g., more than 30% of total astaxanthin exist in the *Z*-form in human plasma (Coral-Hinostroza et al., 2004; Østerlie et al., 2000).

Several studies have shown that *Z*-isomers of astaxanthin have higher bioavailability (Coral-Hinostroza et al., 2004; Yang et al., 2017a) and antioxidant capacity than the all-*E*-isomer (Yanget al., 2017b; Liu and Osawa, 2007). It indicates that the intake of astaxanthin *Z*-isomers rather than the (all-*E*)-isomer is preferable for health reasons. Thus, it is important to understand the methods for *Z*-isomerization of astaxanthin and the types of functionalities that change following the *Z*-isomerization. The aim of this paper is to systematically summarize the various isomerization methods of astaxanthin and the effects of the isomerization on the functionalities reported so far. Furthermore, the aspects of the analytical method for astaxanthin *Z*-isomers and change in physicochemical properties of astaxanthin by *E*/*Z*-isomerization are also included in this review. Since the changes between functionality and physicochemical properties by *Z*-isomerization of (all-*E*)-astaxanthin should be closely related, understanding and linking of the both are also important.

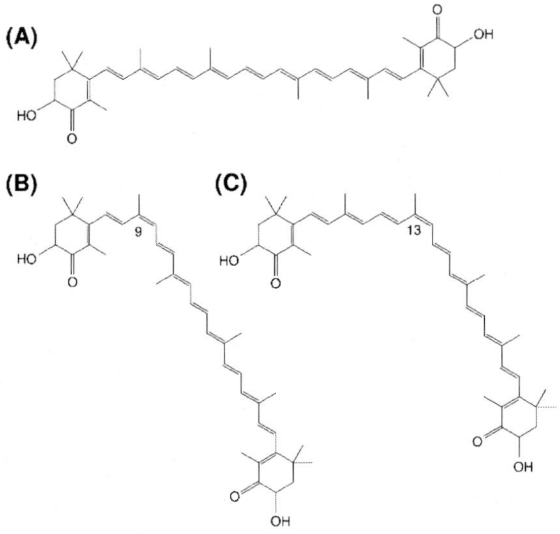

Figure 1. Chemical structures of (A) (all-*E*)-astaxanthin, (B) (9*Z*)-astaxanthin, and (C) (13*Z*)-astaxanthin.

METHOD FOR ANALYZING ASTAXANTHIN ISOMERS

Most studies have used reverse-phase high-performance liquid chromatography (HPLC) with C_{18} (octadecylsilyl silica gel, ODS) column to analyze astaxanthin isomers (Kaga et al., 2018; Yuan and Chen, 1999; Zhao et al., 2005). These studies used the mobile phase consisted of a mixture of methanol, acetonitrile, water, and dichromethane (CH_2Cl_2). That condition could clearly separate (all-*E*)-astaxanthin, (9*Z*)-, and (13*Z*)-

astaxanthin, which are the typical isomers found in human blood (Coral-Hinostroza et al., 2004; Østerlie et al., 2000) and fishes (Bjerkeng et al., 1997; Østerlie et al., 1999). A few studies have conducted the reverse-phase HPLC analysis using a column packed with triacontyl-bonded silica (C_{30}) (Mariutti et al., 2012; Qiu et al., 2012). When using C_{30} column, the analysis time became long compared with using C_{18} column, whereas the separating ability is considerably improved, i.e, multi-*Z*-isomers were separated more clearly. Since astaxanthin isomers have a maximum wavelength around 470 nm (Table 1), astaxanthin isomers were usually measured at a wavelength around 470 nm.

Table 1. Absorption maxima (λ_{max}) and relative intensities of the *Z*-peak (Q-ratio) for geometrical astaxanthin isomers

Compound	λ_{max} (nm)	Q-ratio[a]
(all-*E*)-Astaxanthin	478[b]	–[b]
(9Z)-Astaxanthin	370, 470[b]	0.21[b]
(13Z)-Astaxanthin	370, 468[b]	0.57[b]
(15Z)-Astaxanthin	371, 470[c]	0.66[c]
(9Z,13Z)-Astaxanthin	302, 456[c]	0.22[c]
(9Z,13'Z)-Astaxanthin	301, 460[c]	0.27[c]
(9Z,15Z)-Astaxanthin	324, 459[c]	0.30[c]
(13Z,13'Z)-Astaxanthin	286, 450[c]	0.21[c]
(13Z,15Z)-Astaxanthin	304, 456[c]	0.21[c]

[a] Q-ratio is obtained as the height ratio of the Z-peak to the main absorption peak.
[b] Values were obtained by Yang et al., 2017b.
[c] Values were obtained by Qiu et al., 2012.

For example, Liu and Osawa (2007) and Yuan and Chen (1999) measured astaxanthin isomers at wavelengthes of 471 nm and 480 nm, respectively. Although (all-*E*)-astaxanthin have a main absorption peak around 480 nm, the main absorption peak of astaxanthin *Z*-isomers shift on the side of short wavelength in the range from 450 nm to 470 nm (Table 1) (Qiu et al., 2012; Yang et al., 2017b). Thus, when a sample rich in astaxanthin *Z*-isomers is analyzed by HPLC, it is preferable to set the detection wavelength at around 470 nm, where the differences in molar extinction coefficients among astaxanthin isomers are relatively small, like Liu and Osawa (2007).

In general, astaxanthin isomers which are separated by chromatographies are identified by mass spectrometry (MS) and ^{1}H- and ^{13}C-nuclear magnetic resonance (NMR) (Euglert and Vecchi, 1980; Holtin et al., 2009; Qiu et al., 2012). Moreover, as a simple method, astaxanthin isomers could be identified by its Q-ratio, which was defined as the absorbance ratio of the *Z*-peak to the maximum absorption peak (Table 1). Regardless of astaxanthin, since carotenoid *Z*-isomers have a specific absorption peak around 350 nm, a number of studies related to carotenoids isomers tentatively identified the isomers using Q-ratio (Honda et al., 2015 and 2017b; Li et al., 2012).

Method for *Z*-Isomerization of (All-*E*)-Astaxanthin

To date, several methods for *Z*-isomerization of astaxanthin have been reported, e.g., heat treatment, microwave irradiation, light irradiation, and catalytic treatment (Table 2). Generally, *Z*-isomerization of carotenoids is promoted under dissolved state in oils and organic solvents. Yuan et al. (1999) reported that some organic solvents enhanced *Z*-isomerization of astaxanthin. The *Z*-isomerization promoting effect of organic solvents against astaxanthin were higher in the order of CH_2Cl_2 > chloroform ($CHCl_3$) > the mixture of CH_2Cl_2 and methanol (25:75) > methanol > acetonitrile > acetone > dimethyl sulfoxide. (13*Z*)-Astaxanthin was the main converted isomer in all solvents. Other carotenoids such as lycopene and β-carotene were also promoted *Z*-isomerization in CH_2Cl_2 and $CHCl_3$ (Honda et al., 2014; Sun et al., 2010).

Heat treatment of carotenoids dissolved in oils and organic solvents is the most familiar procedure for promoting the *Z*-isomerization (Holtin et al., 2009; Kaga et al., 2018; Lee et al., 2016; Yang et al., 2015; Zeb and Murkovic, 2011).

Table 2. Summary of representative *Z*-isomerization studies of astaxanthin

Method	Material	Medium solution	Condition	Mainly generated *Z*-isomers	Reference
Heat treatment	Pacific white shrimp	—	Boiling water	(9*Z*), (13*Z*)	Yang et al., 2015
Heat treatment	(all-*E*)-Astaxanthin standard	Olive oil	110 °C	(9*Z*), (13*Z*)	Zab et al., 2011
Heat treatment	(all-*E*)-Astaxanthin standard	CH_2Cl_2	80 °C	(9*Z*), (13*Z*)	Kaga et al., 2018; Honda et al., 2018a
Heat treatment	(all-*E*)-Astaxanthin standard	Dimethyl formamide	150 °C	(9*Z*), (13*Z*), (15*Z*), (9*Z*,13*Z*)	Euglert and Vecchi, 1980
Microwave treatment	Pacific white shrimp	—	600 W	(9*Z*), (13*Z*)	Yang et al., 2015
Microwave treatment	(all-*E*)-Astaxanthin standard	CH_2Cl_2/ethanol	600 W	(9*Z*), (13*Z*)	Zhao et al., 2006
Light irradiation with iodine	(all-*E*)-Astaxanthin standard	Benzene	Daylight fluorescence tube	(9*Z*), (13*Z*), (15*Z*), (9*Z*,13*Z*)	Euglert and Vecchi, 1980
Light irradiation with iodine	(all-*E*)-Astaxanthin standard	CH_2Cl_2	Natural sunlight	(9*Z*), (13*Z*), (15*Z*), (9*Z*,13*Z*)	Qiu et al., 2012
Catalytic treatment	(all-*E*)-Astaxanthin standard	Ethanol	Copper(II) ion	(9*Z*), (13*Z*)	Zhao et al., 2005
Catalytic treatment	(all-*E*)-Astaxanthin standard	CH_2Cl_2/acetonitrile	Calcium ion	(9*Z*), (13*Z*)	Chen et al., 2007

(all-*E*)-Astaxanthin also isomerized to the *Z*-isomers by heating. For example, high purity (all-*E*)-astaxanthin dissolved in refined olive oil was isomerized to the 9*Z*- and 13*Z*-isomers by heating at 110°C (Zeb and Murkovic, 2011). In addition, Kaga et al. (2018) reported that high purity (all-*E*)-astaxanthin isomerized to the 9*Z*- and 13*Z*-isomers by heating in CH_2Cl_2, and the total *Z*-isomer content reached 39.4% at 80°C for 3 h. (9*Z*)- and (13*Z*)-Astaxanthin were mainly produced from the all-*E*-isomer by heat treatment, whereas, in high temperature such as 150°C, the multi-*Z*-isomers such as the 9*Z*,13*Z*- and 9*Z*,15*Z*-isomers increased in considerable quantity (Euglert and Vecchi, 1980).

A few studies reported that microwave irradiation enhanced *Z*-isomerization of (all-*E*)-astaxanthin (Yang et al., 2015; Zhao et al., 2006). Yang et al. (2015) conducted microwave treatment for Pacific white shrimp (*Litopenaeus vannamei*). When treated at 600 W for more than 3 min, a considerable quantity of (all-*E*)-astaxanthin converted to the 9*Z*- and 13*Z*-isomers. Zhao et al. (2006) reported that microwave irradiation induced the *Z*-isomerization, preferentially to the 13*Z*-isomer, of (all-*E*)-astaxanthin dissolved in a mixture of CH_2Cl_2 and ethanol. (all-*E*)-Lycopene dissolved in organic solvents and vegetable oils were also isomerized to the *Z*-isomers by microwave irradiation, and the *Z*-isomerization efficiency was higher than the conventional heating (Honda et al., 2018b; Kessy et al., 2013).

Z-Isomerization of (all-*E*)-carotenoids including astaxanthin by light irradiation in presence of iodine is also well documented. Euglert and Vecchi (1980) reported that light irradiation using daylight fluorescence tubes to (all-*E*)-astaxanthin dissolved in benzene containing iodine enhanced the *Z*-isomerization. When using this method, not only the mono-*Z*-isomers but also the di-*Z*-isomers such as the 9*Z*,13*Z*- and 13*Z*,15*Z*-isomers generated (Euglert and Vecchi, 1980; Qiu et al., 2012). Other carotenoids, e.g., lutein and zeaxanthin, were also promoted *Z*-isomerization by light irradiation in presence of iodine (Updike and Schwartz, 2003). Although no reports are available on astaxanthin, carotenoids such as lycopene and β-carotene were enhanced *Z*-isomerization by light irradiation with chlorophyll *a* (Honda et al., 2014;

Jensen et al., 1982). It is considered that the photosensitized *Z*-isomerization of carotenoids enhanced through the triplet state (Honda et al., 2014). Thus, when carotenoids are isomerized by this method, the selection of an appropriate photosensitizers, which can lead carotenoids to the triplet state, is very important.

A few studies reported that *Z*-isomerization of (all-*E*)-astaxanthin was promoted in the presence of some positive ions (Chen et al., 2007; Zhao et al., 2005). Zhao et al. (2015) reported that the addition of copper(II) chloride to (all-*E*)-astaxanthin solution induced the *Z*-isomerization, and similarly, Chen et al. (2007) confirmed that calcium ion promoted *Z*-isomerization of astaxanthin. Both studies showed that *Z*-isomerization was promoted by the formation of astaxanthin-positive ion complex and the 9*Z*- and 13*Z*-isomers were predominantly generated. Other carotenoids, e.g., lycopene and β-carotene, were also promoted the *Z*-isomerization in the presence of iron(III) chloride and titanium tetrachloride (Honda et al., 2015; Rajendran and Chen, 2007). Those studies proposed the *E*/*Z*-isomerization mechanism of carotenoids using catalysts. Referring to them, the anticipated *Z*-isomerization mechanism of (all-*E*)-astaxanthin by copper(II) chloride is shown below:

$$(\text{Astaxanthin})_E + Cu^{2+} \rightleftharpoons (\text{Astaxanthin}^{\bullet+})_E + Cu^{+} \quad (1)$$

$$(\text{Astaxanthin}^{\bullet+})_E + Cu^{2+} \rightleftharpoons (\text{Astaxanthin}^{2+})_E + Cu^{+} \quad (2)$$

$$(\text{Astaxanthin}^{\bullet+})_E \rightleftharpoons (\text{Astaxanthin}^{\bullet+})_Z \quad (3)$$

$$(\text{Astaxanthin}^{2+})_E \rightleftharpoons (\text{Astaxanthin}^{2+})_Z \quad (4)$$

$$(\text{Astaxanthin}^{2+})_Z + Cu^{+} \rightleftharpoons (\text{Astaxanthin}^{\bullet+})_Z + Cu^{2+} \quad (5)$$

$$(\text{Astaxanthin}^{\bullet+})_Z + Cu^{+} \rightleftharpoons (\text{Astaxanthin})_Z + Cu^{2+} \quad (6)$$

Although there is no evidence about astaxanthin, some other *Z*-isomerization methods for carotenoids were reported, i.e., electrochemical (Gao et al., 1996; Kispert et al., 2004) and ultrasonic irradiation (Carail et al., 2015; Xu and Pan, 2013) methods. Especially, the electrochemical method had high efficiency for *Z*-isomerization of carotenoids, whereas the method was only confirmed for β-carotene, canthaxanthin, and 8′ -apo- β -caroten-8′ -al (Gao et al., 1996; Kispert et al., 2004). Thus, there is still considerable room for development in the isomerization methods for astaxanthin.

EFFECT OF *Z*-ISOMERIZATION OF (ALL-*E*)-ASTAXANTHIN ON THE PHYISICOCHEMICAL PROPERTIES

Several studies confirmed that *Z*-isomerization of carotenoids induced the change in physicochemical properties such as solubility in solvents, crystallinity, melting point, and stability (Hempel et al., 2016; Honda et al., 2017a; Murakami et al., 2017a, 2017b, and 2018). There is only limited evidence but the physicochemical properties of astaxanthin was also changed by the *Z*-isomerization (Honda et al., 2018a; Kaga et al., 2018). Table 3 shows the effect of *Z*-isomer content on the solubility in three organic solvent; ethanol, acetone, and hexane. Regardless of the solvent polarity, as the *Z*-isomer content increased, the solubility of astaxanthin improved, e.g., the solubility in ethanol of astaxanthin containing 63.2% *Z*-isomer is approximately 700 times higher than that of the all-*E*-isomer. The solubilities of lycopene and β-carotene were also improved by the *Z*-isomerization (Honda et al., 2018a; Murakami et al., 2017a and 2017b).

Differential scanning calorimetry (DSC), powder X-ray diffraction (XRD), and scanning electron microscopy (SEM) analyses clearly showed that increasing the *Z*-isomer content of astaxanthin, the melting point was lowered and it was less prone to crystallize and became amorphous (Honda et al., 2018a). (all-*E*)-Astaxanthin molecules can be stabilized via π-π-stacking interactions of conjugated polyene chains, and thus carotenoids show high crystalline properties. However, as the *Z*-isomer content of astaxanthin, enormous steric hindrance occurs, diminishing the potential attractive π-π forces, resulting in the change of melting point and crystallinity (Hempel., et al., 2016; Murakami et al., 2017a). De Bruijn et al. (2016) reported that the molar extinction coefficients of astaxanthin isomers were different among them and were determined in the order of (9*Z*)- > (all-*E*)- > (13*Z*)-astaxanthin. Thus, the color value of astaxanthin isomers should become same older in the above. With its higher molar extinction coefficient than that of (all-*E*)-astaxanthin, formation of (9*Z*)-astaxanthin would partially compensate for the color loss induced by conjugated double bond cleavage in the parental (all-*E*)-astaxanthin. As for the stability of astaxanthin isomers, Kaga et al. (2018) reported that emulsified astaxanthin *Z*-isomers had lower storage stability than the all-*E*-isomer. Also in other carotenoids such as lycopene, the all-*E*-isomer had higher storage stability than the *Z*-isomer against heating and light irradiation (Murakami et al., 2018), and that was also confilmed by computational methods using gaussian software (Honda et al., 2017a).

Table 3. Solubility in organic solvents of astaxanthin containing different *Z*-isomer contents[a]

Solvent	Solubility (mg/L)		
	All-*E*	34.5% *Z*	63.2% *Z*
Ethanol	8.1 ± 0.1	3495.7 ± 187.1	5642.4 ± 53.7
Acetone	155.5 ± 1.6	4545.4 ± 161.0	5714.0 ± 113.0
Hexane	1.3 ± 0.0	1515.4 ± 27.0	1539.0 ± 18.4

[a] Values were obtained by Honda et al., 2018a.

Table 4. Summary of differences in physicochemical properties between (all-*E*)-astaxanthin and the *Z*-isomers[a]

Solubility	Crystallinity	Melting point	Color value	Stability
(*E*) < (*Z*)	(*E*) > (*Z*)	(*E*) > (*Z*)	(9*Z*) > (*E*) > (13*Z*)	(*E*) > (*Z*)

[a] (*E*), (all-*E*)-astaxanthin; (*Z*), *Z*-isomers of astaxanthin; (9*Z*), (9*Z*)-astaxanthin; (13*Z*), (13*Z*)-astaxanthin.

The differences in physicochemical properties between (all-*E*)-astaxanthin and the *Z*-isomer are summarized in Table 4. These differences should have close relationship with the changes in the bioavailability and functionality by the *Z*-isomerization of astaxanthin. In terms of bioavailability, generally, carotenoids uptake into intestinal mucosal cells is aided by the formation of bile acid misselles. Hence, since astaxanthin *Z*-isomers have higher solubility in the micells than the all-*E*-isomers, they are preferentially incorporated into enterocytes and showed a higher bioavailability (Boileau et al., 1999; Coral-Hinostroza et al., 2004; Desmarchelier and Borel 2017; Yang et al., 2017a).

In recent years, utilizing the change in physicochemical properties of carotenoids with the *Z*-isomerization, improvement of the processing efficiency is actively studied. For example, when lycopene in tomatoes and gac (*Momordica cochinchinensis* Spreng.) was thermally *Z*-isomerized before the solvent extraction, the extraction efficiency was greatly improved (Honda et al., 2017c and 2018c). In addition, the emulsification efficiency of β-carotene and micronization efficiency of lycopene were also improved by the *Z*-isomerization pre-treatment (Kodama et al., 2018; Ono et al., 2018). However, to my best knowledge, there is no report about improvement of processing efficiency of astaxanthin by the *Z*-isomerization pre-treatment. Hence, development of research in this field using astaxanthin is expected in the future.

Effect of *Z*-Isomerization of (All-*E*)-Astaxanthin on the Bioavailability and Anitioxidant Activity

Some papers have addressed that *Z*-isomerization of astaxanthin induced the changes in bioavailability (Table 5). Oral-dosing tests for a fich, Rainbow trout (*Oncorhynchus mykiss*), showed that (all-*E*)-astaxanthin have higher bioavailability than the *Z*-isomers (Bjerkeng et al., 1997; Østerlie et al., 1999). For example, Bjerkeng et al. (1997) reported that when pelleted diets rich in astaxanthin having different *Z*-isomer content (97% of all-*E*-isomers and 64% all-*E*-isomer) were fed to rainbow trout (*Oncorhynchus mykiss*) for 69 days, flesh carotenoid concentration of the trout fed (all-*E*)-astaxanthin tended to be higher than in trout fed the astaxanthin rich in the *Z*-isomers (10.0 and 8.6 mg/kg, respectively). On the other hand, the *in vitro* tests using a simulated digestion model and human intestinal Caco-2 cells and human oral-dosing tests showed a greater potential for bioavailability of the *Z*-isomers (Coral-Hinostroza et al., 2004; Østerlie et al., 2000; Yang et al., 2017a). Yang et al. (2017a) reported that (13*Z*)-astaxanthin exibited higher bioaccesibility than the all-*E*-isomer in a simulated digestion model, and (9*Z*)-astaxanthin showed higher cellular-transport efficiency than the all-*E*-isomer in Caco-2 cell monolayers. In human, when the astaxanthin source consisted of 74% (all-*E*)-, 9% (9*Z*)-, 17% (13*Z*)-astaxanthin was ingested, (9*Z*)- and (13*Z*)-astaxanthin was selectively accumulated in plasma (Østerlie et al., 2000). Thus, it is conceivable that intake of astaxanthin *Z*-isomers could be preferable human because of their good bioavailability. As for other carotenoids, ample studies have addressed that *Z*-isomers of lycopene had higher bioavailability than the all-*E*-isomers (Boileau et al., 1999; Cooperstone et al., 2015; Failla et al., 2008; Unlu et al., 2007), whereas *Z*-isomers of β-carotene were less bioavailable than the all-*E*-isomers (Deming et al., 2002; During et al., 2002; Stahl et al., 1995).

Although according to the assay method employed, many studies indicated that *Z*-isomerization of astaxanthin enhanced the antioxidant activity (Table 5). For example, antioxidant enzyme-activity, diphenylpicrylhydrazyl (DPPH) radical scavenging, oxygen radical-absorption capacity (ORAC), photochemiluminescence (PLC), and lipid-peroxidation assays showed higher antioxidant activities of astaxanthin *Z*-isomers compared with the all-*E*-isomers (Liu and Osawa, 2007; Yang et al., 2017a; Yang et al., 2017b). On the other hand, when evaluated by a cellular antioxidant actibity (CAA) assay, the antioxidant activities were higher in the order of (13*Z*)- > (all-*E*)- > (9*Z*)-astaxanthin (Yang et al., 2017b). Other carotenoids *Z*-isomers, e.g., lycopene, cantaxanthin, and lutein, also showed higher antioxidant activity than the *Z*-isomers in the several assay methods such as DPPH, ORAC, ferric reducing antioxidant power (FRAP), and trolox equivalent antioxidant capacities (TEAC) assays

(Böhm et al., 2002; Müller et al., 2011; Venugopalan et al., 2013; Yang et al., 2018).

To my best knowledge, the changes in functionalities of astaxanthin by the *Z*-isomerization were reported only about bioavailability and antioxidant activity. However, in other carotenoids such as β-carotene, cantaxanthin, and fucoxanthin, the *Z*-isomerization improved anti-atherogenesis, pro-apoptotic, and anti-cancer activities, respectively (Harari et al., 2013; Nakazawa et al., 2009; Relevy et al., 2015; Venugopalan et al., 2009). Thus, further progress in this research area using astaxanthin is expected.

Table 5. Summary of the effects of astaxanthin *Z*-isomerization on the bioavailability and functionality

Evaluation	Evaluation method	Advantage[a]	Reference
Bioavailability/ bioaccessibility	Rainbow trout (*Oncorhynchus mykiss*) oral-dosing test	(*E*) > (*Z*)	Bjerkeng et al., 1997; Østerlie et al., 1999
	Human oral-dosing test	(*E*) < (*Z*)	Østerlie et al., 2000
	Human oral-dosing test	(*E*) < (*Z*)	Coral-Hinostroza et al., 2004
	Digestion model and Caco-2 cells	(*E*) < (*Z*)	Yang et al., 2017a
Antioxidant activity	DPPH and lipid-peroxidation assays	(*E*) < (*Z*)	Liu and Osawa, 2007
	DPPH, ORAC, and PLC assays	(*E*) < (*Z*)	Yang et al., 2017b
	CAA assay	(13*Z*) > (*E*) > (9*Z*)	Yang et al., 2017b
	Antioxidant enzyme-activity assay	(*E*) < (*Z*)	Yang et al., 2017a

[a] (*E*), (all-*E*)-astaxanthin; (*Z*), *Z*-isomers of astaxanthin; (9*Z*), (9*Z*)-astaxanthin; (13*Z*), (13*Z*)-astaxanthin.

Conclusion

This chapter summarized methods for HPLC analysis of astaxanthin *Z*-isomers and the *Z*-isomerization, and the effects of the *Z*-isomerization on the physicochemical properties (solubility in solvents, crystallinity, melting point, color value, and stability) and fuctionalities (bioavailability and antioxidant activity). These information are usuful for development of practically feasible method for *Z*-isomerization of (all-*E*)-astaxanthin and for discovery of new functions of the *Z*-isomers.

Z-Isomerization of astaxanthin might offer positive effects for the bioavailability and antioxidant activity. However, as far as I know, the *Z*-isomer-rich products have not appeared in the market. That would be because the *Z*-isomerization of astaxanthin in an industrial scal is difficult and the *Z*-isomers are unstable. In the future, I hope that the above ploblems will be solved, and products rich in astaxanthin *Z*-isomers such as supplements and drinks will be sold.

Acknowledgments

The authors are grateful to Prof. Motonobu Goto (Department of Materials Process Engineering, Nagoya University), Prof. Chitoshi Kitamura, Dr. Yoshinori Inoue, and Dr. Munenori Takehara (Department of Materials Science, The University of Shiga Prefecture), and Hiroyuki Ueda, Dr. Tetsuya Fukaya, and Ryota Takemura (Innovation Division, Kagome Co., Ltd.) for their kind help and constructive suggestions.

References

Ambati, R. R., Phang, S. M., Ravi, S., Aswathanarayana, R. G. (2014). Astaxanthin: sources, extraction, stability, biological activities and its commercial applications—a review. *Marine Drugs*, 12 (1), 128-152.

Bjerkeng, B., Følling, M., Lagocki, S., Storebakken, T., Olli, J. J., Alsted, N. (1997). Bioavailability of all-*E*-astaxanthin and *Z*-isomers of astaxanthin in rainbow trout (*Oncorhynchus mykiss*). *Aquaculture*, 157 (1-2), 63-82.

Böhm, V., Puspitasari-Nienaber, N. L., Ferruzzi, M. G., Schwartz, S. J. (2002). Trolox equivalent antioxidant capacity of different geometrical isomers of α-carotene, β-carotene, lycopene, and zeaxanthin. *Journal of Agricultural and Food Chemistry*, 50 (1), 221-226.

Boileau, A. C., Merchen, N. R., Wasson, K., Atkinson, C. A., Erdman, J. W., Jr (1999). *Cis*-lycopene is more bioavailable than *trans*-lycopene *in vitro* and *in vivo* in lymph-cannulated ferrets. *The Journal of Nutrition*, 129 (6), 1176-1181.

Carail, M., Fabiano-Tixier, A. S., Meullemiestre, A., Chemat, F., Caris-Veyrat, C. (2015). Effects of high power ultrasound on all-*E*-β-carotene, newly formed compounds analysis by ultra-high-performance liquid chromatography–tandem mass spectrometry. *Ultrasonics Sonochemistry*, 26, 200-209.

Chen, C. S., Wu, S. H., Wu, Y. Y., Fang, J. M., Wu, T. H. (2007). Properties of astaxanthin/Ca^{2+} complex formation in the deceleration of cis/trans isomerization. *Organic Letters*, 9 (16), 2985-2988.

Cooperstone, J. L., Ralston, R. A., Riedl, K. M., Haufe, T. C., Schweiggert, R. M., King, S. A., Timmers, C. D., Francis, D. M., Lesinski, G. B., Clinton, S. K., Schwartz, S. J. (2015). Enhanced bioavailability of lycopene when consumed as *cis* - isomers from *tangerine* compared to red tomato juice, a randomized, cross - over clinical trial. *Molecular Nutrition & Food Research*, 59 (4), 658-669.

Coral-Hinostroza, G. N., Ytrestøyl, T., Ruyter, B., Bjerkeng, B. (2004). Plasma appearance of unesterified astaxanthin geometrical *E*/*Z* and optical *R*/*S* isomers in men given single doses of a mixture of optical 3 and 3′ *R*/*S* isomers of astaxanthin fatty acyl diesters. *Comparative Biochemistry and Physiology Part C: Toxicology & Pharmacology*, 139 (1-3), 99-110.

De Bruijn, W. J., Weesepoel, Y., Vincken, J. P., Gruppen, H. (2016). Fatty acids attached to all-*trans*-astaxanthin alter its *cis-trans* equilibrium, and consequently its stability, upon light-accelerated autoxidation. *Food Chemistry*, 194, 1108-1115.

Deming, D. M., Teixeira, S. R., Erdman, J. W., Jr (2002). All-*trans* β-carotene appears to be more bioavailable than 9-*cis* or 13-*cis* β-carotene in gerbils given single oral doses of each isomer. *The Journal of Nutrition*, 132 (9), 2700-2708.

Desmarchelier, C., Borel, P. (2017). Overview of carotenoid bioavailability determinants: From dietary factors to host genetic variations. *Trends in Food Science & Technology*, 69, 270-280.

During, A., Hussain, M. M., Morel, D. W., Harrison, E. H. (2002). Carotenoid uptake and secretion by CaCo-2 cells: β-carotene isomer selectivity and carotenoid interactions. *Journal of Lipid Research*, 43 (7), 1086-1095.

Euglert, G., Vecchi, M. (1980). *trans*/*cis* Isomerization of astaxanthin diacetate/isolation by HPLC and identification by ^{1}H - NMR spectroscopy of three mono - *cis* - and six di - *cis* - Isomers. *Helvetica Chimica Acta*, 63 (6), 1711-1718.

Failla, M. L., Chitchumroonchokchai, C., Ishida, B. K. (2008). *In vitro* micellarization and intestinal cell uptake of *cis* isomers of lycopene exceed those of all-*trans* lycopene. *The Journal of Nutrition*, 138 (3), 482-486.

Gao, G., Wei, C. C., Jeevarajan, A. S., Kispert, L. D. (1996). Geometrical isomerization of carotenoids mediated by cation radical/dication formation. *The Journal of Physical Chemistry*, 100 (13), 5362-5366.

Harari, A., Abecassis, R., Relevi, N., Levi, Z., Ben-Amotz, A., Kamari, Y., Harats, A., Shaish, A. (2013). Prevention of atherosclerosis progression by 9-*cis*-β-carotene rich alga *Dunaliella* in apoE-deficient mice. *BioMed Research International*, 2013, 169517 (1-7).

Hempel, J., Schädle, C. N., Leptihn, S., Carle, R., Schweiggert, R. M. (2016). Structure related aggregation behavior of carotenoids and carotenoid esters. *Journal of Photochemistry and Photobiology A: Chemistry*, 317, 161-174.

Holtin, K., Kuehnle, M., Rehbein, J., Schuler, P., Nicholson, G., Albert, K. (2009). Determination of astaxanthin and astaxanthin esters in the microalgae *Haematococcus pluvialis* by LC-(APCI) MS and characterization of predominant carotenoid isomers by NMR spectroscopy. *Analytical and Bioanalytical Chemistry*, 395, 1613-1622.

Honda, M., Igami, H., Kawana, T., Hayashi, K., Takehara, M., Inoue, Y., Kitamura, C. (2014). Photosensitized *E*/*Z* isomerization of (all-*E*)-lycopene aiming at practical applications. *Journal of Agricultural and Food Chemistry*, 62 (47), 11353-11356.

Honda, M., Kawana, T., Takehara, M., Inoue, Y. (2015). Enhanced *E*/*Z* isomerization of (all-*E*)-lycopene by employing iron(III) chloride as a catalyst. *Journal of Food Science*, 80 (7), C1453-C1459.

Honda, M., Kodama, T., Kageyama, H., Hibino, T., Wahyudiono., Kanda, H., Goto, M. (2018a). Enhanced solubility and reduced crystallinity of carotenoids, β - carotene and astaxanthin, by *Z* - isomerization. *European Journal of Lipid Science and Technology*, 1800191 (1-8).

Honda, M., Kudo, T., Kuwa, T., Higashiura, T., Fukaya, T., Inoue, Y., Kitamura, C., Takehara, M. (2017a). Isolation and spectral characterization of thermally generated multi-*Z*-isomers of lycopene and the theoretically preferred pathway to di-*Z*-isomers. *Bioscience, Biotechnology, and Biochemistry*, 81 (2), 365-371.

Honda, M., Murakami, K., Watanabe, Y., Higashiura, T., Fukaya, T., Wahyudiono, Kanda, H., Goto, M. (2017b). The *E*/*Z* isomer ratio of lycopene in foods and effect of heating with edible oils and fats on isomerization of (all-*E*)-lycopene. *European Journal of Lipid Science and Technology*, 119 (8), 1600389 (1-9).

Honda, M., Sato, H., Takehara, M., Inoue, Y., Kitamura, C., Takemura, R., Fukaya, T., Wahyudiono, Kanda, H., Goto, M. (2018b). Microwave - accelerated *Z* - isomerization of (all - *E*)-lycopene in tomato oleoresin and enhancement of the conversion by vegetable oils containing disulfide compounds. *European Journal of Lipid Science and Technology*, 120 (7), 1800060 (1-9).

Honda, M., Watanabe, Y., Murakami, K., Hoang, N. N., Wahyudiono, Kanda, H., Goto, M. (2018c). Enhanced lycopene extraction from gac (*Momordica cochinchinensis* Spreng.) by the *Z* - isomerization induced with microwave irradiation pre - treatment. *European Journal of Lipid Science and Technology*, 120 (2), 1700293 (1-8).

Honda, M., Watanabe, Y., Murakami, K., Takemura, R., Fukaya, T., Kanda, H., Goto, M. (2017c). Thermal isomerization pre-treatment to improve lycopene extraction from tomato pulp. *LWT-Food Science and Technology*, 86, 69-75.

Jensen, N. H., Nielsen, A. B., Wilbrandt, R. (1982). Chlorophyll *a* sensitized *trans-cis* photoisomerization of *all-trans*-β-carotene. *Journal of the American Chemical Society*, 104 (22), 6117-6119.

Kaga, K., Honda, M., Adachi, T., Honjo, Wahyudiono, M., Kanda, H., Goto, M. (2018). Nanoparticle formation of PVP/astaxanthin inclusion complex by solution-enhanced dispersion by supercritical fluids (SEDS): Effect of PVP and astaxanthin *Z*-isomer content. *The Journal of Supercritical Fluids*, 136, 44-51.

Kessy, H. N., Zhang, L., Zhang, H. (2013). Lycopene (Z)-isomers enrichment and separation. *International Journal of Food Science & Technology*, 48 (10), 2050-2056.

Kispert, L. D., Konovalova, T., Gao, Y. (2004). Carotenoid radical cations and dications: EPR, optical, and electrochemical studies. *Archives of Biochemistry and Biophysics*, 430 (1), 49-60.

Kodama, T., Honda, M., Takemura, R., Fukaya, T., Uemori, C., Wahyudiono, Kanda, H., Goto, M. (2018). Effect of the *Z*-isomer content on nanoparticle production of lycopene using solution-enhanced dispersion by supercritical fluids (SEDS). *The Journal of Supercritical Fluids*, 133, 291-296.

Lee, Y. R., Li, X., Row, K. H. (2016). Isomer separation of *trans*-astaxanthin, 9-*cis*-astaxanthin and 13-*cis*-astaxanthin by ligand exchange chromatography. *Asian Journal of Chemistry*, 28 (6), 1185-1190.

Li, H., Deng, Z., Liu, R., Loewen, S., Tsao, R. (2012). Ultra-performance liquid chromatographic separation of geometric isomers of carotenoids and antioxidant activities of 20 tomato cultivars and breeding lines. *Food Chemistry*, 132 (1), 508-517.

Liu, X., Osawa, T. (2007). *Cis* astaxanthin and especially 9-*cis* astaxanthin exhibits a higher antioxidant activity *in vitro* compared to the all-*trans* isomer. *Biochemical and Biophysical Research Communications*, 357 (1), 187-193.

Mariutti, L. R., Pereira, D. M., Mercadante, A. Z., Valentão, P., Teixeira, N., Andrade, P. B. (2012). Further insights on the carotenoid profile of the echinoderm *Marthasterias glacialis* L. *Marine Drugs*, 10 (7), 1498-1510.

Müller, L., Goupy, P., Fröhlich, K., Dangles, O., Caris-Veyrat, C., Böhm, V. (2011). Comparative study on antioxidant activity of lycopene (*Z*)-isomers in different assays. *Journal of Agricultural and Food Chemistry*, 59 (9), 4504-4511.

Murakami, K., Honda, M., Takemura, R., Fukaya, T., Kubota, M., Wahyudiono, Kanda, H., Goto, M. (2017a). The thermal *Z*-isomerization-induced change in solubility and physical properties of (all-*E*)-lycopene. *Biochemical and Biophysical Research Communications*, 491 (2), 317-322.

Murakami, K., Honda, M., Takemura, R., Fukaya, T., Wahyudiono, Kanda, H., Goto, M. (2018). Effect of thermal treatment and light irradiation on the stability of lycopene with high *Z*-isomers content. *Food Chemistry*, 250, 253-258.

Murakami, K., Honda, M., Wahyudiono, Kanda, H., Goto, M. (2017b). Thermal isomerization of (all-*E*)-lycopene and separation of the *Z*-isomers by using a low boiling solvent: Dimethyl ether. *Separation Science and Technology*, 52 (16), 2573-2582.

Nakazawa, Y., Sashima, T., Hosokawa, M., Miyashita, K. (2009). Comparative evaluation of growth inhibitory effect of stereoisomers of fucoxanthin in human cancer cell lines. *Journal of Functional Foods*, 1 (1), 88-97.

Ono, M., Honda, M., Wahyudiono, Yasuda, K., Kanda, H., Goto, M. (2018). Production of β-carotene nanosuspensions using supercritical CO_2 and improvement of its efficiency by *Z*-isomerization pre-treatment. *The Journal of Supercritical Fluids*, 138, 124-131.

Østerlie, M., Bjerkeng, B., Liaaen-Jensen, S. (1999). Accumulation of astaxanthin all-*E*, 9*Z* and 13*Z* geometrical isomers and 3 and 3′ *RS* optical isomers in rainbow trout (*Oncorhynchus mykiss*) is selective. *The Journal of Nutrition*, 129 (2), 391-398.

Østerlie, M., Bjerkeng, B., Liaaen-Jensen, S. (2000). Plasma appearance and distribution of astaxanthin *E*/*Z* and *R*/*S* isomers in plasma lipoproteins of men after single dose administration of astaxanthin. *The Journal of Nutritional Biochemistry*, 11 (10), 482-490.

Ouchi, A., Aizawa, K., Iwasaki, Y., Inakuma, T., Terao, J., Nagaoka, S. I., Mukai, K. (2010). Kinetic study of the quenching reaction of singlet oxygen by carotenoids and food extracts in solution. Development of a singlet oxygen absorption capacity (SOAC) assay method. *Journal of Agricultural and Food Chemistry*, 58 (18), 9967-9978.

Qiu, D., Wu, Y. C., Zhu, W. L., Yin, H., Yi, L. T. (2012). Identification of geometrical isomers and comparison of different isomeric samples of astaxanthin. *Journal of Food Science*, 77 (9), C934-C940.

Rajendran, V., Chen, B. H. (2007). Isomerization of β-carotene by titanium tetrachloride catalyst. *Journal of Chemical Sciences*, 119 (3), 253-258.

Relevy, N. Z., Rühl, R., Harari, A., Grosskopf, I., Barshack, I., Ben-Amotz, A., Nir, U., Gottieb, H., Kamari., Y., Harats, D., Shaish, A. (2015). 9-*cis*-β-carotene inhibits atherosclerosis development in female LDLR-/-Mice. *Functional Foods in Health and Disease*, 5 (2), 67-79.

Stahl, W., Schwarz, W., von Laar, J., Sies, H. (1995). All-*trans* β-carotene preferentially accumulates in human chylomicrons and very low density lipoproteins compared with the 9-*cis* geometrical isomer. *The Journal of Nutrition*, 125 (8), 2128-2133.

Sun, Y., Ma, G., Ye, X., Kakuda, Y., Meng, R. (2010). Stability of all-*trans*-β-carotene under ultrasound treatment in a model system: effects of different factors, kinetics and newly formed compounds. *Ultrasonics Sonochemistry*, 17 (4), 654-661.

Unlu, N. Z., Bohn, T., Francis, D. M., Nagaraja, H. N., Clinton, S. K., Schwartz, S. J. (2007). Lycopene from heat-induced *cis*-isomer-rich tomato sauce is more bioavailable than from all-*trans*-rich tomato sauce in human subjects. *British Journal of Nutrition*, 98 (1), 140-146.

Updike, A. A., Schwartz, S. J. (2003). Thermal processing of vegetables increases cis isomers of lutein and zeaxanthin. *Journal of Agricultural and Food Chemistry*, 51 (21), 6184-6190.

Venugopalan, V., Tripathi, S. K., Nahar, P., Saradhi, P. P., Das, R. H., Gautam, H. K. (2013). Characterization of canthaxanthin isomers isolated from a new soil *Dietzia* sp. and their antioxidant activities. *J. Microbiol. Biotechnol*, 23 (2), 237-245.

Venugopalan, V., Verma, N., Gautam, H. K., Saradhi, P. P., Das, R. H. (2009). 9-*cis*-Canthaxanthin exhibits higher pro-apoptotic activity than all-*trans*-canthaxanthin isomer in THP-1 macrophage cells. *Free Radical Research*, 43 (2), 100-105.

Visioli, F., Artaria, C. (2017). Astaxanthin in cardiovascular health and disease: mechanisms of action, therapeutic merits, and knowledge gaps. *Food & Function*, 8 (1), 39-63.

Xu, Y., Pan, S. (2013). Effects of various factors of ultrasonic treatment on the extraction yield of all-*trans*-lycopene from red grapefruit (*Citrus paradise* Macf.). *Ultrasonics Sonochemistry*, 20 (4), 1026-1032.

Yang, C., Fischer, M., Kirby, C., Liu, R., Zhu, H., Zhang, H., Chen, Y., Sun, Y., Zhang, L., Tsao, R. (2018). Bioaccessibility, cellular uptake and transport of luteins and assessment of their antioxidant activities. *Food Chemistry*, 249, 66-76.

Yang, C., Zhang, H., Liu, R., Zhu, H., Zhang, L., Tsao, R. (2017a). Bioaccessibility, cellular uptake, and transport of astaxanthin isomers and their antioxidative effects in human intestinal epithelial Caco-2 cells. *Journal of Agricultural and Food Chemistry*, 65 (47), 10223-10232.

Yang, C., Zhang, L., Zhang, H., Sun, Q., Liu, R., Li, J., Wu, L., Tsao, R. (2017b). Rapid and efficient conversion of all-*E*-astaxanthin to 9*Z*- and 13*Z*-isomers and assessment of their stability and antioxidant activities. *Journal of Agricultural and Food Chemistry*, 65 (4), 818-826.

Yang, S., Zhou, Q., Yang, L., Xue, Y., Xu, J., Xue, C. (2015). Effect of thermal processing on astaxanthin and astaxanthin esters in pacific white shrimp *Litopenaeus vannamei*. *Journal of Oleo Science*, 64 (3), 243-253.

Yuan, J. P., Chen, F. (1999). Isomerization of *trans*-astaxanthin to *cis*-isomers in organic solvents. *Journal of Agricultural and Food Chemistry*, 47 (9), 3656-3660.

Zeb, A., Murkovic, M. (2011). Carotenoids and triacylglycerols interactions during thermal oxidation of refined olive oil. *Food Chemistry*, 127 (4), 1584-1593.

Zhang, L., Wang, H. (2015). Multiple mechanisms of anti-cancer effects exerted by astaxanthin. *Marine Drugs*, 13 (7), 4310-4330.

Zhao, L., Chen, F., Zhao, G., Wang, Z., Liao, X., Hu, X. (2005). Isomerization of *trans*-astaxanthin induced by copper(II) ion in ethanol. *Journal of Agricultural and Food Chemistry*, 53 (24), 9620-9623.

Zhao, L., Zhao, G., Chen, F., Wang, Z., Wu, J., Hu, X. (2006). Different effects of microwave and ultrasound on the stability of (all-*E*)-astaxanthin. *Journal of Agricultural and Food Chemistry*, 54 (21), 8346-8351.

INDEX

A

B

C

D

E

F

G

H

I

K

L

M

N

O

P

R

S

T

U

V

W

X

Z

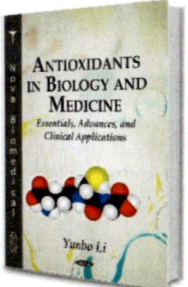

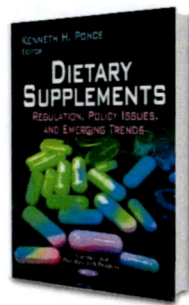